Deliciously Healthy
Fertility

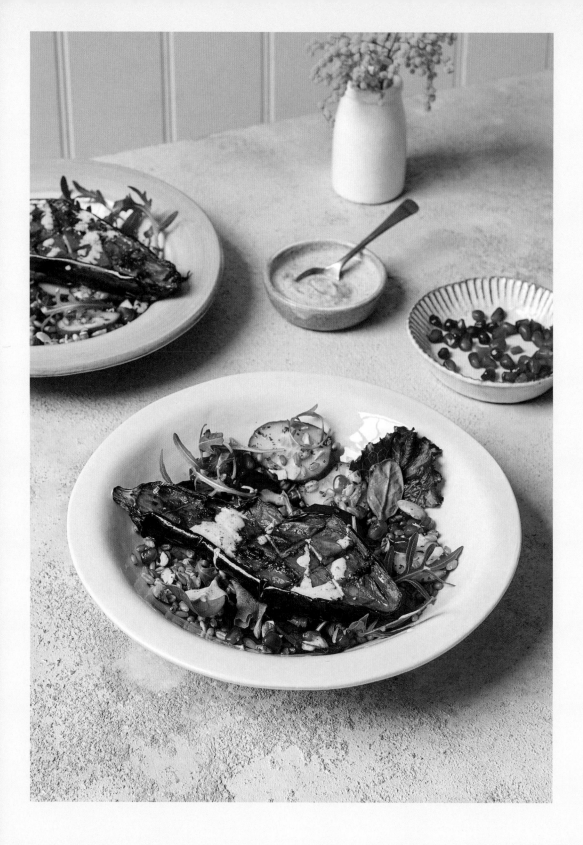

Deliciously Healthy

Fertility

Nutrition and recipes to help you conceive

RO HUNTRISS

Contents

Preface

The importance of a mom-to-be's diet in pregnancy is well understood—a baby needs nutrients to grow and develop and it obtains these from its mother's diet. However, the importance of a preconception diet—for women and men—is often overlooked, yet it can not only influence your baby's health but also play a significant role in optimizing fertility.

Diet and lifestyle can't solve every fertility issue, but they can help regulate menstrual cycles, improve egg and sperm quality, influence implantation, and reduce the risk of miscarriage. As awareness of how diet impacts fertility remains low, I am so glad to be sharing this science with you and explaining how to apply it practically to your own life.

I began to explore the field of fertility nutrition when I became acutely aware of the lack of support and trustworthy dietary advice available to women and men trying to conceive, or planning to conceive in the future. I realized that many people were eager to make changes to their diet and lifestyle to support their fertility but didn't know what changes to make and whether they would make a difference. They were looking for guidance and support. I wanted to help, and with my background as a dietitian with masters' degrees in both Advanced Nutrition and Clinical Research and a huge passion for this area, I was confident I could.

Being 35 myself at the time of writing this book, I'm also aware of the number of women who are having children later in life for a variety of different reasons. We know that as we age, biology isn't on our side, but nutrition and lifestyle can be. Being equipped with knowledge of how fertility can be optimized through diet and how we live can help many couples who are trying to conceive later in life.

I dedicated years to reviewing hundreds, if not thousands, of research papers related to nutrition, lifestyle, and fertility and saw that there really were significant associations between what women and men ate, the supplements they took, their lifestyles, and their fertility outcomes. I started sharing this evidence-based information on my Instagram page @fertility.dietitian.uk and began to support couples through their journeys to conception and beyond. I really began to see the power of this science in action—how it has changed and created lives.

This book aims to make trustworthy nutritional advice accessible to all the couples who need it. It discusses the basics of human reproduction, examines the issues that couples may face, and looks at how the nutrients in their diets, coupled with their lifestyles, can help solve different pieces of the fertility puzzle for women and men. The second half of the book sees the science of fertility nutrition translated into more than 60 recipes so you can be confident that what you're eating supports your journey and goals, while understanding why these recipes can help.

Thank you for choosing this book—I truly hope that it supports and inspires you on your own unique journey.

Ro Huntriss

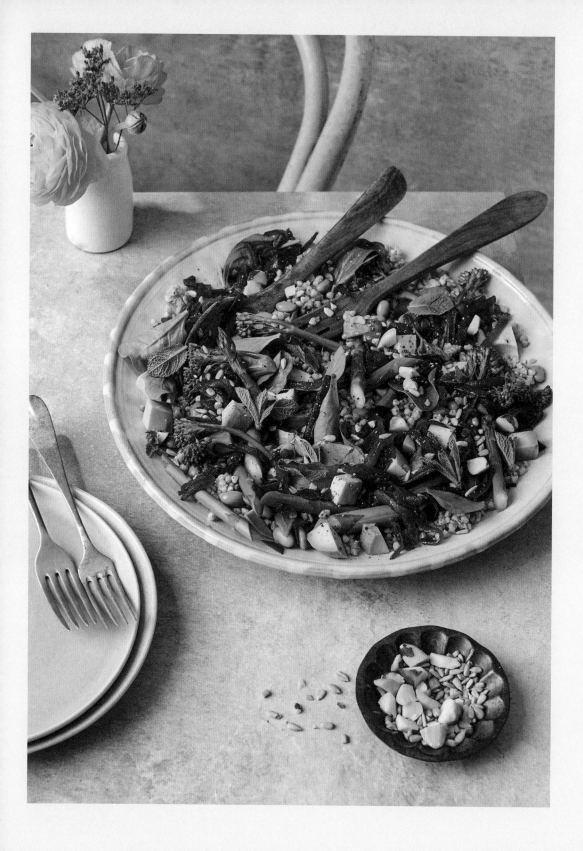

A guide
to fertility

Understanding the fundamentals of the reproductive processes, as well as the factors both within and beyond your control that can affect your chances of conceiving, can help you take steps where possible to enhance your own fertility. The following section explains what helps and hinders fertility and explores how your diet and lifestyle can have a significant impact on your chances of conception and a successful pregnancy.

Understanding women's reproductive cycles

Women are born with all their eggs, in the form of immature oocytes (see p.22), which stay dormant in the ovaries until puberty, at around the age of 12. Each month, one dominant follicle (sometimes more) releases a mature egg during ovulation, ready for fertilization. The process by which an egg matures is closely controlled by your hormones during the menstrual cycle.

How your hormones govern the menstrual cycle

Every month, the cascade of hormonal changes, illustrated opposite, occurs in your body to prepare you for a possible pregnancy. This monthly cycle begins on the first day of your period and lasts until the day before your next period. During each cycle, an egg released from one of your ovaries could—if all the conditions are right—be fertilized by a sperm, form an embryo, and develop into a pregnancy. In some cases, more than one follicle may release an egg, increasing the chance of having twins, or more.

If an egg is fertilized, it divides rapidly to form an embryo. This travels down the Fallopian tube to your uterus, where it's ready to implant in the uterine lining. If the embryo implants successfully, your body releases a hormone called human chorionic gonadotropin (hCG). This hormone is detected in pregnancy tests to signal that your pregnancy has begun. The interplay between reproductive hormones—progesterone, estrogen, follicle stimulating hormone (FSH), and luteinizing hormone (LH)—is crucial for a healthy, functioning menstrual cycle and conception. If your hormones become unbalanced, this can affect their control of the menstrual cycle and your ability to conceive successfully (see pp.18–19).

It takes around three months for an immature oocyte to mature into an egg that is ready to be released at ovulation. This makes the three months before conception a valuable opportunity to influence the quality of your eggs through your diet and lifestyle (see pp.32–81).

Your menstrual cycle hormones and fertile "window"

Your cycle comprises two phases: the follicular phase starts on the first day of your period and lasts until ovulation. The luteal phase begins once an egg is released and ends either with your next period or a fertilized egg, ready for implantation. As sperm can live for up to five days, your most fertile window is the five days before ovulation and up to 24 hours after an egg is released (see p.12). The graph below is based on an average cycle length, but variations are common (see p.12).

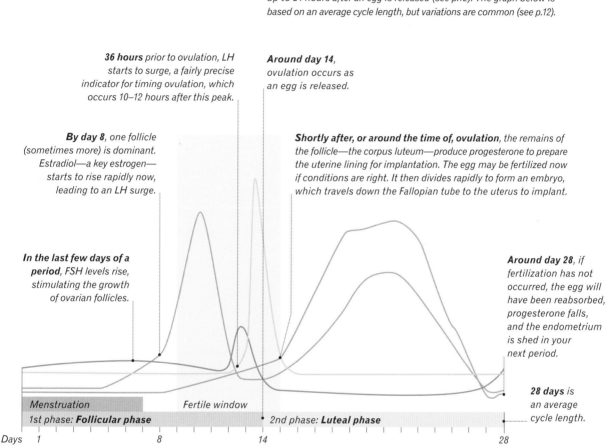

36 hours prior to ovulation, LH starts to surge, a fairly precise indicator for timing ovulation, which occurs 10–12 hours after this peak.

Around day 14, ovulation occurs as an egg is released.

By day 8, one follicle (sometimes more) is dominant. Estradiol—a key estrogen— starts to rise rapidly now, leading to an LH surge.

Shortly after, or around the time of, ovulation, the remains of the follicle—the corpus luteum—produce progesterone to prepare the uterine lining for implantation. The egg may be fertilized now if conditions are right. It then divides rapidly to form an embryo, which travels down the Fallopian tube to the uterus to implant.

In the last few days of a period, FSH levels rise, stimulating the growth of ovarian follicles.

Around day 28, if fertilization has not occurred, the egg will have been reabsorbed, progesterone falls, and the endometrium is shed in your next period.

Menstruation

Fertile window

1st phase: **Follicular phase**

2nd phase: **Luteal phase**

28 days is an average cycle length.

Days   1   8   14   28

Progesterone, a vital female hormone, prepares your uterus for implantation by a fertilized egg.
• Once an egg is fertilized, progesterone stimulates the growth of blood vessels that supply the uterine lining—the endometrium—to help implantation. It also stimulates the endometrium to secrete nutrients and proteins called growth factors to aid tissue growth.
• After implantation, signals sent to the ovaries increase progesterone levels. Adequate progesterone is needed to maintain the uterine lining, making this hormone crucial for the survival of early pregnancy.

Estrogen is a key reproductive hormone. Estradiol is one of the three main natural estrogens.
• Estrogen helps control the menstrual cycle.
• It prepares the uterus for pregnancy by stimulating the lining to grow and thicken, ready to accept a fertilized egg—or embryo.

FSH (follicle stimulating hormone)
• This stimulates the growth of ovarian follicles, one—sometimes more—of which will release an egg when you ovulate.

LH (luteinizing hormone)
• The surge in this hormone that occurs toward the end of the follicular phase of your menstrual cycle triggers ovulation.

Monitoring your own menstrual cycle

A typical menstrual cycle is around 28 days long, with ovulation occurring on day 14. However, cycles can vary widely between women and regular cycles can be anywhere from 21 to 35 days—occasionally longer. On average, women ovulate between days 11 and 21 of a cycle. When you ovulate will depend on the length of your own cycle among other factors. If your cycle is regular, this is a good indicator that your reproductive system is working normally. If your cycle varies in length, this doesn't necessarily indicate a problem, but it can be worth discussing with your health-care provider. Charting your cycle with an app or calendar can help you be more in tune with your body and understand your own unique cycle, which in turn can support your chance of conceiving.

Identifying when your body ovulates

Ovulation doesn't always happen on the same day each month, so if you're trying to conceive, the advice is to have sexual intercourse every two to three days for a good chance of conception. One of the ways to further increase your chance of becoming pregnant is to identify when ovulation occurs in a particular month. Your most fertile time is around the five days before to the day following ovulation (see p.11), so having regular sex in this window of opportunity is likely to give you the best chance of becoming pregnant.

An ovulation test—which detects the hormonal changes involved in ovulation—can help you figure out when you're ovulating. Some tests check for the surge in luteinizing hormone (LH) just before ovulation (see p.11), signaling that an egg will be released in the next 12 to 36 hours. Others test for the preovulatory rises in estrogen and LH to help identify a longer fertile window, as oestrogen rises a few days earlier.. Ovulation tests can be a helpful tool, especially if you have regular cycles. However, with conditions such as polycystic ovary syndrome (PCOS; see p.18), or for women who have irregular periods or are taking certain medications, they can be less useful.

Looking out for the physiological changes, discussed opposite, that occur in your body around the time of ovulation is another way to identify the most fertile part of your cycle. If some of these changes don't occur, such as a temperature rise or there's an absence of cervical mucus, this may indicate an ovulatory issue (see p.19). Talk to your health-care provider if you're concerned, who can decide if investigations may be worthwhile.

READING THE SIGNS OF OVULATION

Monitor changes in your cervical mucus

Changes to the texture, amount, color, and consistency of cervical mucus occur throughout your cycle. Controlled by hormones, these changes can be a helpful indicator of ovulation. After menstruation, you may have dry days with no mucus. As estrogen rises, mucus starts to develop that can be thick, white, and fibrous, making it very hard for sperm to pass through. Around ovulation, mucus becomes profuse, clear, stretchy, and slippery—similar to raw egg white. This is "fertile" mucus as sperm can pass through it and survive in it for up to five days. After ovulation, mucus thickens, becomes cloudy, and on some days may be absent, indicating that your most fertile time has passed.

Try tracking your basal body temperature

The release of progesterone after ovulation (see p.11) causes your core body temperature to rise slightly. A digital thermometer can help you chart your basal body temperature—the body's lowest temperature at rest—daily to identify when ovulation has occurred. A rise of 0.4°F that remains steady for three days or more indicates ovulation may have occurred. This increase is sustained for the luteal phase of the cycle, until your next period. Charting your temperature over a few months can help you spot patterns so you can better understand your cycle and when you tend to ovulate (or flag an ovulatory problem, see p.19), in turn supporting your chances of becoming pregnant.

Notice an increased sex drive

A rise in estrogen in the days leading up to ovulation often results in an increased libido—one indicator that you're in your most fertile window.

Consider checking the position of your cervix

During ovulation, your cervix rises higher in the vagina and feels soft, like your ear lobe. You can check its position yourself by consulting reputable online sources. It's best to check and record its position daily during your cycle so you can spot and monitor changes.

Look out for ovulation pain

Some women get a one-sided pain in their lower abdomen when they ovulate. It's not entirely clear why this occurs, but some experts believe it may be caused by fluid released when an egg breaks through the ovary wall, irritating nerves. It's usually harmless and can help support other ovulatory indicators. If pain concerns you, talk to your health-care provider.

Understanding men's reproductive systems

Hormones play a key role in the male reproductive system. Together, hormones, the production of healthy sperm, and the mechanics of ejaculation all contribute to men's fertility.

The role of hormones in male reproduction

As with women, reproduction in men is closely controlled by hormones. Reductions or imbalances in any of the following hormones can affect sex drive, erection, ejaculation, sperm production, and fertility (see p.21).

- **Testosterone** is the main hormone produced in the testes. It regulates spermatogenesis—the process by which the body makes sperm (see opposite). It's needed for the vital processes involved in sperm production, including the division and reshaping of sperm cells as they transform into mature sperm. It's also important for libido, erection, and ejaculation.

Ideal sperm parameters

The diagram below sets out optimal sperm measures and characteristics from the World Health Organization (WHO). These are considered ideal levels that are most likely to lead to fertilization.

Volume per ejaculation

1.5–5ml volume of semen per ejaculate is the normal range.

Sperm count

Over *39 million* sperm per ejaculate is within normal parameters.

Motility (movement)

At least 40% motile sperm per ejaculate is desirable, with 32% of these having "progressive" motility (see opposite).

More than *15 million* sperm per ml is considered normal.

Concentration

Ideally, there are at least *58% live sperm* per ejaculate.

Vitality (live sperm)

Although the proportion sounds small, at least *4% regular-shaped sperm* is seen as normal.

Morphology (shape)

○ Sperm measures

● Sperm characteristics

- **Luteinizing hormone (LH) and follicle stimulating hormone (FSH)** are produced by the pituitary gland. LH controls the production of testosterone and FSH is involved in controlling sperm production.
- **Oxytocin**, often referred to as the "love hormone," helps regulate male orgasm and ejaculation. At ejaculation, a burst of oxytocin stimulates contractions in the male reproductive tract, in turn aiding sperm release.

Sperm production and ejaculation

Sperm is produced daily in the testes, and mature sperm is stored in the epididymis, a long, coiled tube that transports sperm from the testes prior to ejaculation. It takes around 74 days for sperm to develop in the testes and mature in the epididymis—the sperm regeneration cycle. Continuous production means that sperm are always ready for ejaculation. Where sperm aren't ejaculated, the cells die and are then reabsorbed into the body. Problems with ejaculation and sperm can impact fertility (see p.21).

Sperm count, concentration, volume, vitality, motility (movement), and morphology (shape) are all used to measure sperm health (see opposite).

- **Sperm count** is the number of sperm per ejaculate. A low count reduces the chances of natural conception; however, unless sperm count is zero, conception isn't impossible.
- **Sperm concentration** is a significant factor in sperm health. Millions of sperm start the journey from the ejaculate to the egg, but millions die on the way. A good sperm concentration increases the likelihood that one sperm will successfully complete the journey and fertilize an egg.
- **Sperm volume** is important and an adequate amount is required to carry sperm into the female reproductive tract. However, low sperm volume may not impair fertility if other sperm markers are strong.
- **Sperm vitality** is the percentage of live sperm in an ejaculate. The more live sperm, the better the chance that one will fertilize an egg.
- **Motility (how sperm move)** can determine whether sperm reach an egg. Sperm that swim in mostly straight lines or large circles—referred to as having "progressive motility"—are optimal.
- **Morphology (shape)** is part of the assessment of sperm health, with normal sperm having an oval head and a long tail.

Exploring fertility problems

The World Health Organization (WHO) defines infertility as the failure to become pregnant after 12 months or more of regular unprotected sex. However, the term "infertility" does not mean that a couple can't or won't conceive in the future.

Understanding the terms

If you and/or your partner decide to undergo fertility investigations, being familiar with the terms that health-care providers use can be helpful. "Primary infertility" is where a woman who has never conceived has a problem conceiving. "Secondary infertility" is where a woman has had one or more pregnancies in the past but is struggling to conceive again. In around one in four couples experiencing issues, the cause for the problem isn't identified in either partner, referred to as "unexplained infertility."

Where fertility issues stem from

Much emphasis for fertility problems is placed on women, but men play an equal role in the fertility equation (see opposite). Women can experience issues for a variety of reasons. Ovulatory issues are the most common, or there may be other hormone-related issues or problems with the mechanics of reproduction (see pp.18–21). Men may encounter problems if they have one or more sperm abnormalities (see p.21) and/or they're unable to deliver semen efficiently into the vagina. This may happen, for example, if there's a problem with sperm or a problem with sexual function, such as low libido or erection or ejaculation issues. Testicular swellings known as varicoceles may also cause fertility problems.

When expert help may be needed

If you've been trying to conceive for more than a year, the advice is to consult your medical health-care provider, who may suggest investigations to try to identify a cause. For women over the age of 35, it's best to seek

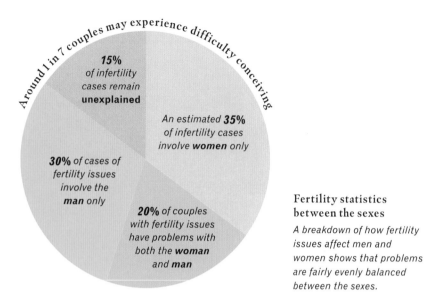

Around 1 in 7 couples may experience difficulty conceiving

15%
*of infertility
cases remain*
unexplained

An estimated **35%**
*of infertility cases
involve* **women** *only*

30% *of cases of
fertility issues
involve the*
man *only*

20% *of couples
with fertility issues
have problems with
both the* **woman**
and **man**

**Fertility statistics
between the sexes**
*A breakdown of how fertility
issues affect men and
women shows that problems
are fairly evenly balanced
between the sexes.*

advice after six months of trying to conceive. Bear in mind that signs that
your body is struggling to conceive may be silent and the only indicator
may be not conceiving successfully. For other couples, issues may be
apparent. If you experience any of the signs below, this doesn't necessarily
mean there's a problem, but if you're also having trouble conceiving, you
may wish to discuss any concerns you have with your health-care provider.

For women, the following may be caused by a fertility issue:
• Heavy, long, or painful periods.
• Irregular or absent periods and/or ovulation.
• An absence of fertile cervical mucus (see p.13).
• Facial hair, acne, or unexplained weight gain, which could
  indicate a hormonal imbalance.
• Pain during sex.
For men, the following may indicate a fertility concern:
• Erectile dysfunction.
• Ejaculation issues.
• Changes in the testicles.

Why fertility problems may arise

Hormonal imbalances, some autoimmune conditions, mechanical problems, and abnormal sperm parameters can all impact fertility. Your diet and lifestyle choices (see pp.32–81) can often make a measurable difference to some of these issues; however, some will require medical intervention.

Hormone-related and autoimmune problems

If couples experience fertility problems, one of the first things that might be checked is hormone levels. Our hormones are crucial for reproduction and an imbalance can affect our chances of conception. Often, treatment and medication can help regulate hormones and, in turn, the menstrual cycle. Some autoimmune conditions such as celiac disease can also affect fertility. Learning to manage these conditions helps support your fertility.

• **Polycystic ovary syndrome (PCOS)** is a leading cause of fertility issues in women. Symptoms such as irregular or absent periods; fluid-filled sacs, or follicles, on the ovaries; and excess male hormones (androgens) can suggest PCOS and investigations can confirm a diagnosis. Many sufferers are resistant to insulin (see p.52), which controls blood sugar levels. Extra insulin is made to compensate, causing the ovaries to overproduce testosterone. The hormonal imbalances—which cause symptoms such as thinning hair, excess body hair, oily skin, acne, and weight gain—can impact fertility. PCOS is often associated with a high BMI but is also seen in those with a healthy BMI, known as "lean PCOS." As well as medication and supplements, diet and lifestyle (see below) can improve symptoms significantly and limit the impact on fertility.

Managing PCOS through diet and lifestyle

This illustration summarizes key dietary and lifestyle recommendations for PCOS sufferers. Pages 76–77 outline the exercise guidelines that are suggested to help manage PCOS.

Do

Diet Moderate your carb intake, choosing low GI carbs; eat plenty of protein (opt for lean meat or plant-based); and include healthy fats in your diet. Lifestyle Incorporate vigorous activity and resistance training. Aim for a healthy weight.

Don't

Diet Avoid a high carb diet and protein-free meals. Reduce your sugar and saturated fat intake. Lifestyle Avoid a sedentary lifestyle.

- **An overactive or underactive thyroid** can cause hormone imbalances. Low levels of thyroid hormones (hypothyroidism) in women can lead to anovulation (see below); low progesterone, which can affect implantation; and other imbalances, impacting ovulation and menstruation. High levels of thyroid hormones (hyperthyroidism) in women can lead to light or irregular periods and reduced conception rates. Hyperthyroidism can affect men, too. Up to 70 percent of men with fertility issues with this condition report problems such as decreased libido, erectile dysfunction, and premature ejaculation. It has also been linked to reduced sperm quality. Medication can restore reproductive function in both women and men.
- **Diabetes** is characterized by high blood glucose (sugar) levels. The hormone insulin is released to control blood sugar (see p.52). If high blood sugar is chronic, the body may become less sensitive to insulin, known as insulin resistance. As a result, more insulin is produced, which can unbalance hormones. Diabetes can disrupt menstruation, and high blood glucose levels increase the risk of miscarriage. In men, diabetes can lead to erectile dysfunction, low testosterone, and reduced sperm quality. Maintaining a healthy weight, being active, eating healthily, and taking medication if required, helps control blood glucose and balance hormones.
- **Cushing's syndrome**, most common in women, is an overproduction of the stress hormone cortisol, causing symptoms such as excess abdominal and chest fat, fatty deposits on the neck or upper back, a rounded face, and purple stretch marks. High cortisol levels also affect the ovaries, leading to irregular cycles or an absence of periods. While this condition can resolve without treatment, medication may be needed to help manage it.
- **Anovulation** is when your ovary doesn't release an egg during a cycle, though there may still be a bleed if the uterine lining has thickened. Occasional anovulation isn't uncommon and is usually not a concern. However, factors such as high or low BMI; hormonal imbalances caused by PCOS; pituitary gland issues; hypothyroidism; and high levels of prolactin—which inhibits FSH, interfering with egg development—can cause chronic anovulation. Irregular or absent periods; very heavy or light periods; a lack of cervical mucus; and, if you're tracking it, no rise in basal body temperature (see p.13) can indicate anovulation. If you've missed three or more periods and aren't pregnant, talk to your health-care provider about possible treatment options.

- **Celiac disease** is an autoimmune condition where the immune system attacks the body's tissues if gluten—a protein in wheat, barley, and rye—is eaten. In women, it's linked to anovulation (see p.19), reduced pregnancy rates, and higher miscarriage rates. In men, it may be associated with testicular problems and changes in sperm morphology (shape) and motility. Sticking to a gluten-free diet helps to manage celiac disease and minimize related fertility issues (see p.50).

Problems with the mechanics of reproduction

Both women's and men's fertility can be impacted by a physical problem with the reproductive organs or system. Being aware of an issue can help you explore your options for conception.

- **Blocked, damaged, or scarred Fallopian tubes** impact fertility. If a Fallopian tube—the thin tube that runs from each ovary to the uterus—is blocked, a released egg may be unable to meet sperm to be fertilized, create an embryo, and reach the uterus. A blockage in one tube reduces fertility as each ovary tends to release an egg on alternating months. If both tubes are blocked, no eggs can reach the uterus and IVF is required. Damaged or scarred tubes increase the risk of an ectopic pregnancy, when a fertilized egg implants outside of the womb, usually in a tube. Unfortunately, this type of pregnancy isn't viable and needs to be removed. Damage, scarring, or blockages have a number of causes, including untreated pelvic inflammatory disease (PID; which can result from a sexually transmitted infection), endometriosis, abdominal surgery, or fibroids. If investigations uncover a problem with your Fallopian tubes, surgery may be considered, and IVF can offer an alternative way forward to conception and pregnancy.

- **Uterine scarring** can be caused by a condition called Asherman's syndrome, which can result from surgery, inflammation, or infection. Scarring affects the blood flow to the endometrium, reducing the chance of implantation. Symptoms can include pelvic pain, light or no periods, recurrent miscarriage, or a failure to conceive. Surgery can be carried out to improve the chances of implantation and pregnancy.

- **Uterine fibroids and polyps**—noncancerous uterine growths—affect around one in three women. Often these are symptomless, but they can cause heavy or painful periods, abdominal pain, frequent urination, and constipation and may impact fertility, for example, by blocking implantation. Their growth is linked to estrogen, and they're associated with obesity, which increases estrogen levels. If they become problematic, medication or surgery to remove them may be discussed.

- **Damaged or undescended testes** can affect the quality of the semen stored in them. Infection, testicular cancer or surgery, a congenital defect, or an injury can all result in damage. Fertility procedures such as sperm extraction and intracytoplasmic sperm injection (ICSI)—where sperm is injected directly into an egg—may be suggested to aid conception.
- **Varicoceles**—an enlargement of the veins in the scrotum, the loose bag of skin that holds the testes—sometimes affect sperm quality. However, two-thirds of men with a varicocele have no difficulty fathering a child. Surgery can correct a varicocele where there is a fertility issue.
- **Ejaculation problems**—the inability to ejaculate semen efficiently— make it harder for sperm to reach an egg. Problems can be caused by a range of factors, including prostate and thyroid issues, recreational drug use, medication, age, and conditions such as diabetes, spinal cord injuries, and multiple sclerosis. Depression, stress, relationship problems, trauma, and anxiety around sexual performance can also have an impact. In some cases, medication, surgery, or talking therapies such as cognitive behavioral therapy (CBT), that connect thoughts to behaviors, can help.

How sperm quality can affect fertility

The health of the sperm in each ejaculate can impact fertility if it falls outside the normal, healthy parameters discussed on pages 14–15. As well as looking at sperm vitality, volume, count, and concentration, a sperm analysis will also measure sperm motility (how sperm move) and morphology (what sperm look like). If sperm can't travel in straight lines, if they move in small circles (non-progressive), or can't travel at all (immotile), this can affect fertility; while head or tail defects can make it harder for sperm to reach and fertilize an egg. Sperm DNA damage can also decrease the chance of creating a viable embryo and increase the risk of miscarriage.

Looking at age and fertility

As we get older, our fertility naturally reduces. However, for women, the effects of age on fertility can be seen much earlier than for men, and age has a larger impact on women's overall chances of conception.

How age affects women's fertility

Women are born with one to two million follicles, or immature eggs (oocytes), that have the potential to develop into a mature egg. By the age of 32, around 12 percent of your prebirth reserve remains, and by the age of 40, only 3 percent. This is known as your ovarian reserve. A test to check for a glycoprotein—anti-müllerian hormone (AMH)—produced by follicles, helps assess reserve; low levels indicate a reduced reserve. For accuracy, this is done alongside a hormone profile and antral folllicle count (AFC) scan. The results can help women make decisions about their fertility journey. Encouragingly, couples can have successful pregnancies, natural and assisted, even when AMH levels are low.

Egg quality also declines with age. As an immature oocyte matures, it goes through a process of cell division. During this process, older eggs are more likely to develop DNA errors that can lead to genetic abnormalities in the egg, reducing pregnancy chances and increasing the risk of miscarriage. Egg quality is also influenced by oxidative stress. We all have some level of oxidative stress, caused by free radicals—molecules that can harm our bodies. Poor diet, charred or overly browned food, excess weight, alcohol, smoking, pollution, and pesticides can increase oxidative stress, and levels in our bodies also rise as we age. This is why some women who may not be ready to conceive until later in life may choose to freeze their eggs when younger to preserve egg quality.

Thinking about your reproductive life span

Recent research estimates that women's average reproductive life span is 37.1 years of age, increased from a previous estimate of 35 years of age.

More and more women are having children in their 30s, and even 40s, than before. At menopause, which typically occurs between the ages of 45 and 55, though can be earlier, menstruation stops and women cease to be fertile.

It is difficult to predict each person's reproductive life span. Generally, the earlier you have children, the fewer fertility risks you are likely to encounter. If circumstances mean that you can control when to start trying for a family, the advice is to try before the age of 35, when ovarian reserve drops considerably. If this is not possible for you, optimizing your diet and lifestyle (see pp.32–81) can promote the quality and quantity of your eggs.

The effect of age on men's fertility

Men can produce new sperm throughout their lifetime and father a child into old age. Although the "biological clock" is less critical for men, their fertility does decline with age, with studies suggesting that sperm quality starts to drop from age 40. Increased age has been linked to reduced production and volume of sperm, reduced sperm numbers, reduced motility (movement), fewer normal-shaped sperm (morphology), and an increase in sperm DNA damage, in turn, reducing the likelihood of conception. Older men also have an increased risk of premature ejaculation.

In addition, men's libido decreases with age, and health concerns that are more common in older people, such as obesity, high blood pressure, and type 2 diabetes, can often affect men's fertility.

Chances of couples conceiving naturally within a year based on the woman's age

Couples in which the woman is under 30 years old

85%

Couples in which the woman is 30 years old

75%

Couples in which the woman is 35 years old

66%

Couples in which the woman is 40 years old

44%

Age and conception rates
This chart shows the chance of conceiving naturally within a year where couples are trying, based on the woman's age. At the age of 35, ovarian reserve starts to decline more noticeably and the chance of conception reduces. By age 40, the chance is almost half of what it was below the age of 30.

Enhancing your fertility

Several fertility risk factors are within our control. What and how much you eat, your lifestyle, and your levels of stress (see p.80) can all impact fertility. Understanding how to manage these areas of your life will help to optimize your chances of conception.

The link between weight and fertility

There is a well-established link between weight and fertility. When we think about weight in the context of fertility, this refers generally to the amount of fat we carry because this can influence conception. It's important to bear in mind that fat is essential for our bodies to perform many key functions (see p.54). It is the amount of body fat we have that can be significant, with both too little and too much body fat potentially impacting fertility.

How excess weight can affect fertility

It's reassuring to know that many women and men with a raised BMI (see below) do successfully conceive. However, a raised BMI can reduce your chances of conception, or mean it can take a bit longer to conceive.

BMI and fertility
A healthy BMI for all ages and sexes is between 18.5 and 24.9. For women, a BMI of above 19 is advised to support ovulation, and guidelines suggest that maintaining a BMI below 30 may reduce time to pregnancy and improve the outcomes of fertility treatments.

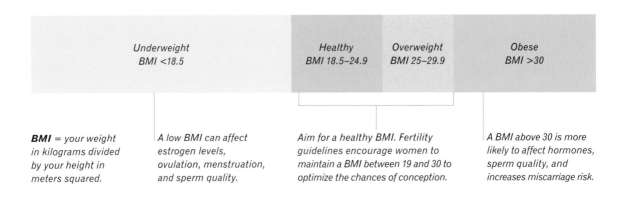

Underweight
BMI <18.5

Healthy
BMI 18.5–24.9

Overweight
BMI 25–29.9

Obese
BMI >30

BMI = *your weight in kilograms divided by your height in meters squared.*

A low BMI can affect estrogen levels, ovulation, menstruation, and sperm quality.

Aim for a healthy BMI. Fertility guidelines encourage women to maintain a BMI between 19 and 30 to optimize the chances of conception.

A BMI above 30 is more likely to affect hormones, sperm quality, and increases miscarriage risk.

For women, excess weight can negatively impact the balance of some reproductive hormones, increasing the level of male hormones (androgens) and levels of estrogen. Obesity is also associated with higher levels of insulin (see p.52)—the hormone that controls blood glucose (sugar) levels—and insulin resistance. As well as making it harder for your body to control blood glucose, this can lead to chronic inflammation and oxidative stress—which can result in cell and tissue damage. Inflammation can impact ovulation, hormone production, and the endometrial lining, while oxidative stress can affect egg quality. All of these hormonal changes can have various effects, including irregular menstrual cycles; irregular, or lack of, ovulation; and issues with the development and quality of eggs, which in turn impact embryo quality. Higher weights have also been linked with implantation problems and an increased miscarriage risk—it's calculated that a BMI over 30 makes the chances of a recurrent miscarriage 1.75 times more likely.

For men, research indicates that being obese can affect sperm quality—lowering volume, sperm count, concentration, vitality, and motility (movement); affecting morphology (shape); and damaging sperm DNA. Carrying excess weight can also lower testosterone levels.

Aside from BMI, waist circumference is key, too, as weight carried on the waist affects metabolic and general health. In couples undergoing fertility treatment, for example, a poor outcome is more likely where men have a higher waist circumference, even if their BMI is normal.

How low weight can affect fertility
Women's fat—adipose tissue—is responsible for producing estrogen. A low BMI can lower estrogen levels. Estrogen plays a key role in regulating the menstrual cycle, in ovulation, and in thickening the uterine lining. If levels are too low, these processes may become irregular or stop entirely.

When low body weight contributes to irregular or absent periods and/or an absence of ovulation, this in turn signals that the body is not in its optimal condition for pregnancy. A low BMI during pregnancy increases the risk of miscarriage, preterm birth, and a low birth weight, so aiming for a healthy prepregnancy weight is very important for you and your baby.

For men, a low BMI has been associated with poor sperm morphology, with a significant number of sperm of abnormal shapes and sizes.

Controlling your weight for fertility

Try these easy-to-implement tips to help you lose or gain weight as needed.

Fertility-friendly tips for losing weight

- Fill half of your plate with vegetables or salad at meals. If the urge to snack strikes, try veggie sticks or fruit for a low-calorie, nutrient-dense option.
- Swap refined carbohydrates, such as white bread, pasta, and rice, for whole grain carbs, such as brown rice, pasta, whole wheat bread, couscous, whole grain quinoa, and buckwheat and oats. These release energy more slowly, helping to satisfy your appetite and reduce cravings.
- Reduce your carbohydrate intake. It's important not to exclude starchy carbs as these are a key source of energy and vital fertility nutrients.
- Up your protein—a filling macronutrient. Choose plant-based proteins over animal-based ones (see p.44) as they're lower in saturated fat and linked to better fertility outcomes. If you eat meat, opt mainly for poultry or leaner cuts.
- Stay hydrated. Aim to drink around eight cups of water or other sugar-free fluid a day (see p.36), ensuring you minimize caffeine. As well as hydrating you, this helps you to manage hunger. Avoid hidden sugars in drinks such as flavored milk.

Fertility-friendly tips for gaining weight

- Incorporate healthy fats—such as extra-virgin olive oil, nuts, seeds, olives, avocados, and high-fat dairy—into every meal and snack.
- Try not to skip meals, even if you don't feel hungry.
- Don't worry about eating too many carbs or occasional "junk" food. This is okay to increase weight, as restoring weight is more important for ovulation.
- Fuel your body appropriately for exercise to avoid a calorie deficit. In addition to meals, snack 30 minutes to an hour before exercise and refuel post-exercise with a food containing carbohydrate and protein.
- Limit vegetables and/or salad to one-third of your plate and ensure you include carbohydrates, fat, and protein. Eating sufficient protein, as well as fat, helps you gain muscle weight.
- Eat four to six smaller meals a day by snacking between meals and having a small supper before bed to help increase your calorie intake.
- Reduce drinks before a meal as these make you feel fuller.

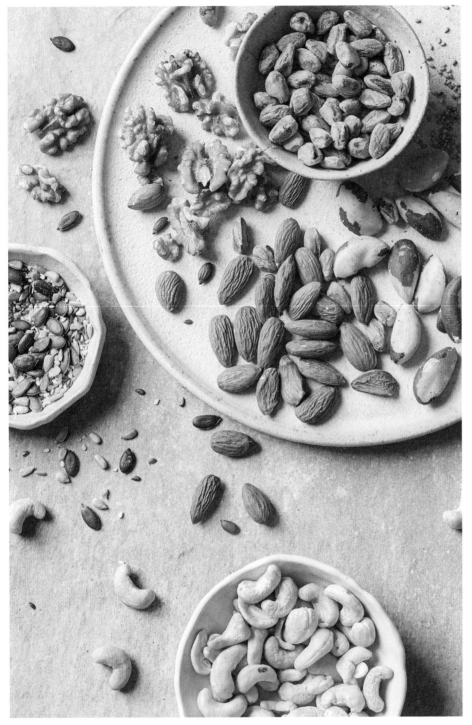

Nuts and seeds make a nutrient-dense snack *that can help you maintain a healthy BMI.*

How other lifestyle factors can affect fertility

As well as eating healthily, exercising sensibly, and managing stress (see pp.32–81), a range of other lifestyle factors can impact your likelihood of becoming pregnant. Making some small lifestyle adjustments can make a big difference to fertility outcomes.

Foods and soft drinks to watch out for

In women, sugar intake, especially from sugar-sweetened drinks, is linked to reduced pregnancy rates. A high sugar intake that leads to high insulin levels (see p.52) can affect women's hormones and how eggs mature. In men, too much sugar may impact sperm concentration and motility. Processed foods up your sugar intake. Evidence on sweeteners is inconclusive, but emerging research suggests that for women, soft diet drinks may affect egg and embryo quality, implantation, and pregnancy rates, while for men, they may impact sperm quality. Saturated fats—found mainly in animal products—should also be limited, and avoid trans fats, found in some processed foods, which can have negative fertility impacts on both sexes.

In early pregnancy, there's usually a short time when a woman doesn't know she has conceived. The advice is to avoid certain foods in pregnancy because of the risk of infections such as salmonella, listeria, and toxoplasmosis, which if contracted increase the risk of miscarriage. If there's a chance you may be pregnant, in particular after ovulation when an egg may have been fertilized, you may wish to follow these guidelines, too. Foods to avoid include unpasteurized cheese and dairy, undercooked meat and shellfish, pâté, and cold meats. Ensure that eggs are pasteurized. Additionally, foods with high levels of vitamin A, such as liver, and foods that contain mercury, such as shark, swordfish, and marlin, should be avoided (and limit tuna consumption). Women should consume 8–12oz seafood per week from choices low in mercury (see p.31).

Thinking about your alcohol consumption

The guideline for women trying to conceive as well as for pregnant women is to not drink any alcohol. If you're experiencing fertility problems, you may feel that an occasional drink is important to help you relax. Understanding the risks can help you make a judgment call. Long-term alcohol intake can disrupt ovulation and lead to irregular periods, and heavy alcohol use (more than 14 units a week) may reduce your number of eggs and is linked to earlier menopause. For women, alcohol also lowers the success rates of fertility treatments. Research suggests that the chance of successful pregnancy reduces as alcohol intake increases. Alcohol also increases your miscarriage risk, with each additional week of even low levels of consumption in the first trimester adding to the risk. Another concern is the effect of alcohol on a fetus; fetal alcohol spectrum disorders (FASD) can affect growth, behavioral and cognitive development, and cause issues such as cleft lip.

For men, drinking more than 14 units a week is linked to lower sperm quality and may contribute to erectile and ejaculatory issues. Low to moderate alcohol consumption doesn't appear to affect male fertility, but studies show that men drinking alcohol in the month prior to fertility treatment can reduce the chance of a live birth, so it's good to take extra care at this time.

Can caffeine affect your fertility?

For women, caffeine is associated with an increased risk of miscarriage and stillbirth. The advice in pregnancy is to keep caffeine intake below 300mg a day and it's good practice to follow the same guidelines when trying to conceive. Some research suggests that even 100mg of caffeine a day could increase the risk of miscarriage, so if you know you have a high risk for miscarriage or have previously miscarried, decreasing this risk by cutting back on caffeine as much as possible could be advantageous.

Studies also suggest that caffeine intake may affect male fertility, possibly by damaging sperm DNA. Therefore it may be advisable for men to limit their caffeine intake to 200–300mg a day.

How much caffeine are you drinking?

Being aware of the amount of caffeine in different drinks helps you calculate your daily intake and moderate it as needed to ensure, for women, that you're consuming below 300mg a day.

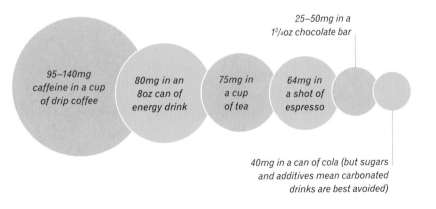

25–50mg in a 1³/₄oz chocolate bar

95–140mg caffeine in a cup of drip coffee

80mg in an 8oz can of energy drink

75mg in a cup of tea

64mg in a shot of espresso

40mg in a can of cola (but sugars and additives mean carbonated drinks are best avoided)

The impact of smoking and recreational drugs on fertility

Smoking lowers conception rates by 10–40 percent. It can also reduce ovarian reserve significantly, affecting natural conception and IVF, and it can disrupt progesterone levels, impacting menstrual cycles and implantation. Studies show that smoking can affect a fertilized egg's journey along a Fallopian tube, increasing conception times and the risk of ectopic pregnancy; while smoking once pregnant increases the risk of miscarriage. With IVF, it can mean the body has a poorer response at a younger age to ovarian stimulation. For men, smoking may lower sperm quantity and quality. Research shows that e-cigarettes can also affect fertility. Even nicotine-free ones have harmful substances such as endocrine disruptors (see below) that affect hormones and reproductive organs.

As well as carrying general health risks, recreational drugs can impact fertility. Marijuana may affect ovulation, and studies suggest that cocaine use can disrupt hormone levels in women. In men, cannabis and anabolic steroids can potentially affect sperm production and function.

Taking medications

Non-steroidal anti-inflammatory drugs (NSAIDs), such as ibuprofen or aspirin, may increase conception times if used over a long period of time. Some prescription drugs can also affect fertility, including antipsychotic drugs; fluid retention drugs; antihistamines; antihypertensives; antibiotics; and antiandrogens. If you take any of these, don't stop but talk to your health-care provider before trying to conceive or if you're experiencing fertility issues.

Other lifestyle practices

Heat can damage sperm. The advice for couples trying to conceive is for men to avoid hot tubs, jacuzzis, or saunas, or taking long hot showers or baths. Men can also avoid wearing tight clothes such as jeans, cycling shorts, or leather trousers, and boxer shorts are preferable to briefs. Electromagnetic radiation from cell phones may also affect sperm. It's best to avoid overusing cell phones or storing them in pants pockets for long periods of time.

Avoiding environmental toxins

Endocrine-disrupting chemicals (EDCs) are compounds that mimic, block, or interfere with hormones in the endocrine system (the organs and glands that make and control hormones). EDCs are found in a range of everyday products, and while research is ongoing, they have been implicated in health concerns, including fertility problems. Studies show that some couples who are struggling to conceive have higher levels of certain chemicals. It's thought that EDCs may contribute to hormone imbalances and irregular cycles, premature ovarian failure, reduced sperm and egg quality, and an increased risk of miscarriage.

Examples of endocrine-disrupting chemicals include bisphenol A (BPA), polychlorinated biphenyls (PCBs), polybrominated diphenyl ethers (PBDEs), phthalates, parabens, and substances known as PFAs. These compounds are found widely in plastics, packaging, toys, clothing, footwear, and personal care products. When thinking about food, bisphenol A (BPA) is especially relevant. This is found in many plastic food storage containers and in artificial resins known as epoxy resins that protect canned foods from contamination. Some evidence suggests that BPA may affect sperm quality, hormone levels, implantation, and impact the number of eggs retrieved in fertility treatments.

Evidence also suggests that exposure to pesticides and herbicides can impact fertility, leading to menstrual cycle disturbances, prolonged conception times, and an increased risk of a miscarriage. Reducing your exposure to EDCs and environmental pollutants to zero is impossible as they are so prevalent, and avoiding them may not be the main focus for all couples trying to conceive. However, if you are struggling to conceive, you may want to consider some of the following lifestyle changes.

- Buy food packaged in cartons rather than cans, or choose BPA-free.
- Wash fruit and vegetables to reduce pesticide and herbicide exposure.
- Reduce prepackaged foods to minimize exposure to plastics.
- Eat oily fish no more than twice a week to limit heavy metal exposure, and reduce fatty meat, which can harbor fat-soluble chemicals and pesticides.
- Drink from glass bottles and cups rather than plastic.
- Do not microwave food in plastic. Transfer food to china or glass bowls covered with a plate or paper towel instead of plastic wrap.
- Avoid air fresheners and heavily perfumed products.
- Open windows to ventilate the home, and use eco cleaning options rather than detergents and cleaning products with strong chemicals.
- Choose paraben-free personal care products.

Your fertility diet

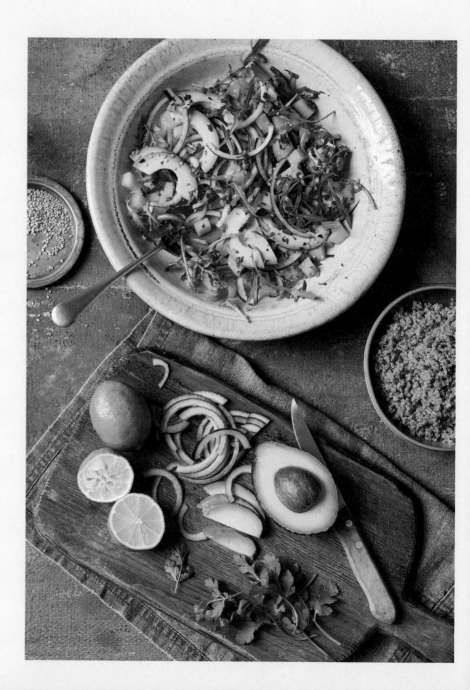

Establishing healthy eating patterns promotes good health and supports well-being throughout your life. At certain times—such as when planning to start a family—what you eat takes on even greater significance.

Once pregnancy is underway, advice on what to eat is abundant. Less discussed is how what you and your partner eat before conception can have a sizable influence on fertility outcomes. During the time it takes for a woman's monthly egg to mature and a man's sperm to develop, you have a valuable nutritional "window" in which to optimize your diet and enhance your chances of conception—whether naturally or via fertility treatments. Paying attention to diet while trying to conceive also ensures that a future pregnancy will have the best possible nutritional start.

The following chapter explains how the foods you eat can influence every aspect of the reproductive journey. Key fertility nutrients for both women and men are discussed—explaining the science behind why these are so helpful, which foods you need to eat to provide them, and which nutrients you need to supplement if dietary sources are low. Advice is also given on which foods can hinder fertility.

Eating to support your fertility is a powerful tool to help you on your journey to parenthood.

Eating for fertility

A balanced, Mediterranean-style diet (see pp.38–41) that's abundant in antioxidants supports all aspects of fertility, from egg and sperm development to a healthy pregnancy.

How your diet can support egg health

The quality of women's eggs is key in determining fertility because this can influence several stages of conception, from the likelihood of an egg being fertilized by a sperm and developing into an embryo to whether that embryo can implant properly into the uterus and the chances that the embryo will continue to develop into a healthy pregnancy.

High levels of oxidative stress, which rise naturally as we age (see p.22), can reduce egg quality. Oxidative stress occurs when there's an imbalance between harmful free radicals and antioxidants—molecules that protect cells against free radicals. A diet high in antioxidants with enough omega-3 (see p.54) helps balance these molecules and support egg quality. A healthy BMI (see p.24) also promotes egg health, as does moderating your intake of sugar, saturated fat, alcohol, and highly processed food.

Your ovarian reserve and ovulation

Women's fertility declines with age as the ovarian reserve—the number of eggs in the ovaries—reduces. Healthy levels of the compound called anti-müllerian hormone (AMH; see p.22) suggest a normal ovarian reserve. Several dietary factors may aid AMH levels. For example, adequate levels of calcium are linked to healthy AMH levels, so including dairy in your diet is beneficial. A high folate intake (see p.61) and good levels of omega-3s (see p.54) are also linked to a healthy ovarian reserve. Premature ovarian insufficiency—when ovarian function reduces before the age of 40—is

Dietary timeline for fertility

Sperm take around 74 days to develop—though this can vary—and an egg takes 90–100 days to mature, ready for ovulation. These time frames provide a window of opportunity to influence egg and sperm quality via your diet.

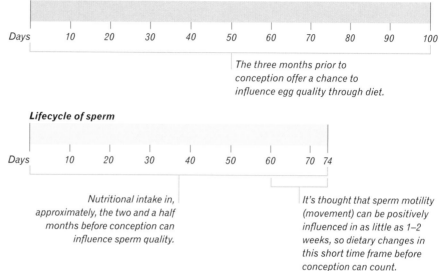

Timeline for an egg to mature

Days   10   20   30   40   50   60   70   80   90   100

The three months prior to conception offer a chance to influence egg quality through diet.

Lifecycle of sperm

Days   10   20   30   40   50   60   70   74

Nutritional intake in, approximately, the two and a half months before conception can influence sperm quality.

It's thought that sperm motility (movement) can be positively influenced in as little as 1–2 weeks, so dietary changes in this short time frame before conception can count.

associated with increased oxidative stress. Research shows that women with this condition who took selenium and vitamin E supplements increased their AMH levels and had a higher antral follicle count (see p.22). Fast foods, a high saturated fat intake (excluding dairy; see p.47), and a high BMI are linked to lower AMH levels and reduced ovarian reserve.

Ovulation is tightly controlled by hormones, and there are many different aspects of diet and lifestyle that can impair or lead to an imbalance in hormone levels, resulting in irregular, or complete lack of, ovulation. Being under- or overweight can influence ovulation, as can nutrient deficiencies, sugar consumption, too little fiber, and the type and amount of fats, carbohydrates, and protein consumed. Pages 44–73 explore the nutrients your body need to optimize ovulation.

Nutrition for healthy sperm

Diet and lifestyle can influence sperm quality both positively and negatively. Eating a Mediterranean-style diet and maintaining a healthy BMI support sperm health. Reducing the intake of red and processed meat, sugar, and saturated fats, avoiding trans fats (see p.54), and moderating alcohol consumption can also benefit sperm quality.

Supporting implantation through your diet

When a fertilized egg travels down the Fallopian tube to implant in the uterus, the uterine lining needs to be thick enough for the egg to implant and for implantation to be sustained. The rise in estrogen in the menstrual cycle (see p.11) helps the uterine lining to thicken and grow, while progesterone maintains the lining and ensures it's receptive to implantation. After implantation, progesterone is still needed to support the growing embryo and insufficient levels can lead to miscarriage. Your nutrient intake supports the action of these hormones, with micronutrients (see pp.60–69) being especially beneficial.

Studies show that folate, vitamin B6, and vitamin C supplements can promote progesterone levels. Vitamin E has antioxidant activity and an anticoagulant effect, which together support the implantation process, possibly by promoting healthy blood flow. A compound called nitric oxide, found in beets and leafy greens (see p.58), dilates blood vessels. This facilitates an oxygen-rich blood flow to the endometrium, which could help implantation. Studies also suggest that supplements of probiotic lactobacillus—found in fermented foods such as kefir and some cottage cheeses—could support implantation.

Healthy omega-3 fats can help reduce inflammation in the body, which supports the process of implantation. For women undergoing IVF, research indicates that a higher intake of whole grains is linked to healthy endometrial thickening, increasing the chances of a successful IVF cycle.

The role of hydration for overall fertility

Alongside your nutrient intake, staying hydrated promotes overall health as well as egg and sperm health and the production of fertile cervical mucus. Aim to drink eight glasses of hydrating fluids a day—more if you exercise or in hot weather. If drinking this amount feels like a struggle, sipping from a bottle of water throughout the day is a good way to keep your fluid intake up. Water is best for hydration. If you like added flavor, try infusing water with fresh produce such as lemon, orange, cucumber, or mint. Other hydrating drinks include decaffeinated tea, coffee, and green tea; herbal teas such as mint, peppermint, or chamomile; and rooibos tea. Avoid drinks with added sugar and limit caffeinated beverages (see p.29).

Sustaining a healthy pregnancy

Sadly, miscarriages are relatively common. In women who know they are pregnant, around one in eight pregnancies end in miscarriage, and it's thought that many more miscarriages occur in women who aren't aware that they're pregnant. The majority of miscarriages are caused by chromosomal or genetic abnormalities that cannot be prevented. If you know you are at an increased risk of miscarriage, you may want to consider dietary measures and supplements that are beneficial in early pregnancy to optimize your chances of sustaining a healthy pregnancy. For example, a higher maternal folate intake is associated with a reduced risk of early pregnancy loss. As well as consuming foods that contain folate (see p.61), taking a daily supplement of 400mcg of folic acid (or more if advised)—or of methylated folate, which is closer to natural folate and may be most suitable where there is a history of recurrent miscarriage—is advised (see p.71). Discuss the best dosage for you with your health-care provider or fertility specialist.

Selenium-rich foods (see p.66) have antioxidant effects thought to be beneficial in early pregnancy, and deficiencies, or low levels, have been associated with a higher risk of miscarriage. Low levels of vitamin B12 (see p.63) are also linked to early pregnancy loss. This vitamin is found only in animal products such as meat, fish, eggs, and dairy, as well as fortified cereals, nutritional yeast, and yeast extracts. If you follow a vegan diet, it's important to take a vitamin B12 supplement. Vitamin D insufficiency may also play a role in early pregnancy loss. If you wish to check your vitamin D levels, discuss this with your health-care provider who may arrange a blood test. As vitamin D can be hard to obtain from diet alone, a supplement of at least 400IU (10mcg) daily is advisable (see p.72).

Maintaining a healthy BMI lowers the risk of miscarriage, with a BMI over 25 associated with a higher risk. It's important to approach weight loss in a fertility-friendly way (see p.26) by maximizing nutritional density in your diet. Following a Mediterranean-style diet will help to ensure this.

If there's a chance you may be pregnant, you might also choose to follow the guidelines on which foods to avoid during pregnancy, on page 28 and minimize your caffeine intake, to ensure that you're not eating anything that may be harmful to your pregnancy or your developing baby.

The Mediterranean diet and fertility

The Mediterranean-style of eating is based on the traditional diet and lifestyle of people in the olive-growing regions of the Mediterranean. Based around fresh and seasonal local ingredients—and an active lifestyle—this way of life has been shown to have a range of impressive benefits for health and well-being. For women and men who are focusing on fertility, adopting a Mediterranean approach also appears to be beneficial.

The benefits of a Mediterranean diet for all

Following the Mediterranean-style of eating has been linked to a whole range of health benefits. The diet has been found to reduce the risk of cardiovascular disease, protect against type 2 diabetes and cognitive decline, and can also be effective in managing weight. The benefits are thanks to its nutrient-rich foods and their protective anti-inflammatory effects. While diets around the world of course reflect different cultures and their associated lifestyles, incorporating elements of the Mediterranean diet, such as eating fish and fresh produce and using vegetable oils, into your own can help you enjoy the associated benefits.

Enhancing your fertility with a Mediterranean diet

The Mediterranean diet is dense in fertility-friendly nutrients such as healthy unsaturated fats, including omega-3; folate and other B vitamins; and a variety of key antioxidants. Numerous studies have highlighted how following this style of eating has favorable effects on women's fertility; while for men, a Mediterranean-inspired diet has been linked to significant improvements in sperm quality, including sperm count and concentration.

The foods that make up a Mediterranean diet generally have a low glycemic index (see pp.52–53), which helps promote healthy blood sugar levels and, in turn, balance insulin levels and other hormones. The diet's anti-inflammatory effects also make it ideal for fertility, in particular for managing inflammatory conditions such as PCOS (see p.18) and endometriosis. Omega-3 fats from fatty fish play a key role in the diet's anti-inflammatory effects, and eating plenty of fresh produce ensures a high intake of antioxidants.

A Mediterranean-style diet also incorporates plenty of nutrient-dense lean protein from sources such as lean meat, fish, and plant-based proteins such as legumes, nuts, and seeds. Opting for leaner protein sources reduces your intake of saturated fat, too much of which is associated with reduced egg and embryo quality. Additionally, increasing your protein intake is thought to support blastocyst development and improve pregnancy rates during IVF (see p.44).

Generally, a Mediterranean diet minimizes your intake of processed foods and red meat, keeping your saturated fat intake at the recommended limits. In contrast, diets that have a lower intake of green vegetables and fruit and a higher intake of fast and processed foods, such as a Western-style diet, have been associated with longer conception times.

How a Mediterranean diet can support fertility treatments

As well as benefits for natural conception, keeping to the principles of a Mediterranean style of eating has been associated with increased success rates in couples undergoing fertility treatments. One study found that a Mediterranean-style diet helped increase embryo yields during IVF treatment, possibly due to either an improved response in the body to ovarian stimulation or improved egg quality.

Another study of Dutch couples found that those who followed a preconception Mediterranean-style diet that was high in vegetable oils, as well as vegetables and fruit, fish, pulses, and whole grains, had a 40 percent increased probability of success in achieving a pregnancy through IVF. In particular, it suggested that it improved the number of embryos yielded in the couples.

Consuming more whole grains has also been linked to a higher chance of implantation and a successful pregnancy in women undergoing IVF.

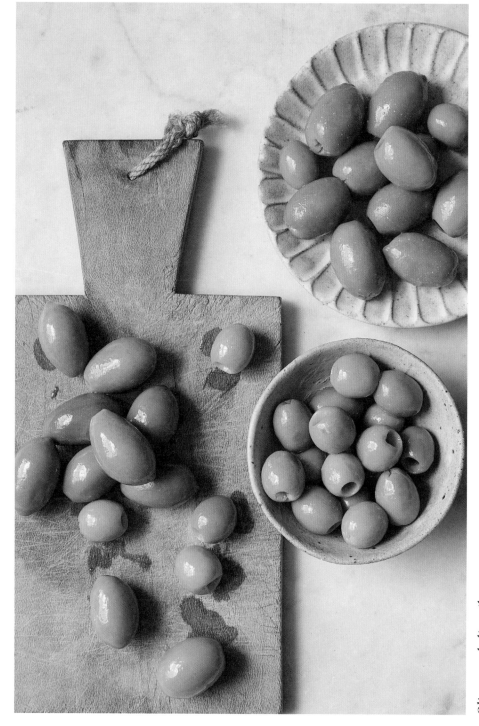

Olives—and olive oil—*provide healthy fats and fertility-supporting antioxidants such as vitamin E.*

Adopting a Mediterranean-style diet

The Mediterranean-style of eating is characterized by a diet rich in fatty fish, vegetables, fruit, nuts, seeds, extra-virgin olive oil, legumes, and whole grains.

- **Enjoy fatty fish**. Consuming 1–2 portions of fatty fish, such as salmon, mackerel, or sardines, every week provides healthy omega-3 fats (see p.54), which have been shown to support fertility.

- **Use olive oil**. Rich in antioxidants such as vitamin E and with a high proportion of monounsaturated fats (see p.54), olive oil supports the reduction of inflammation in the body, an important factor for fertility. Studies looking at a Mediterranean-style of diet high in olive oil have found that this can support embryo development, with improved outcomes for both natural conception and assisted reproductive techniques.

- **Cook with pulses**, such as beans, peas, lentils, chickpeas, and soy beans. A lean source of protein, pulses are also rich in nutrients that support fertility, such as iron and folate, and, importantly, fiber. Plant-based proteins are also thought to support healthy ovulation (see p.44).

- **Opt for whole grains** (see pp.49–50). Aim to make whole grains a regular part of your diet, choosing whole grain bread and pasta, brown rice, oats, quinoa, buckwheat, and whole grain couscous whenever possible. Whole grains are packed full of essential fertility-supporting nutrients such as fiber, B vitamins, and antioxidants.

- **Enjoy different-colored fruits and vegetables** to ensure that you get a wide variety of antioxidants (see pp.56–58), which support many aspects of fertility. Green vegetables especially tend to be high in fertility-supporting folate, so include green vegetables in your meals daily.

- **Eat nuts and seeds**. A source of plant-based protein, these have healthy fats and are rich in antioxidants such as vitamin E, zinc, and selenium. Brazil nuts are a rich source of fertility-promoting selenium. For men, eating nuts is linked to improved sperm quality. Seeds are also a good source of unsaturated fats, including omega-3s, and plant-based protein. Flaxseeds and pumpkin seeds contain lignans—polyphenol compounds associated with shorter conception times—and potent antioxidants such as vitamin E, which support conception.

Following a plant-based diet

A plant-based diet can be interpreted in a number of ways. For some, this is a vegan diet with no animal products, or a vegetarian diet that includes dairy and/or eggs. For others, it's a diet that's made up of predominantly plant-based foods, with just a small amount, or occasional consumption, of animal products such as fish or meat.

A fertility-friendly plant-based diet

Many of the foods recommended for a fertility-supporting diet are plant-based, so if your diet is based around vegetables, fruit, nuts, seeds, whole grains, unsaturated fats, and plant-based protein, it is actually full of fertility-promoting nutrients. However, if you've reduced your consumption of animal-based products, or removed them entirely, there's a risk you could become deficient in certain nutrients important for fertility, which could impact your chances of conception and a healthy pregnancy.

Fortunately, missing nutrients can be provided by supplements and/or you can make food swaps to ensure you're getting the right nutrients. Being aware of which nutrients can be low in a plant-based diet and where to find them can help you plan your meals or replace nutrients with supplements if needed.

- **Protein**, found abundantly in meat, fish, eggs, and milk, is vital for our bodies' processes (see p.44). If you're cutting out or reducing animal proteins, it's essential that you include plenty of plant-based protein alternatives found in soy, pulses, nuts, and quinoa.
- **Omega-3 essential fatty acids** are key for fertility (see p.54). There are several forms of omega-3s: docosahexaenoic acid (DHA), eicosapentaenoic acid (EPA), and alpha-linolenic acid (ALA). EPA and DHA have key reproductive and anti-inflammatory benefits, and the richest source of these is fatty fish, such as salmon, mackerel, and

sardines. In foods with omega-3 ALA, such as flaxseeds, chia seeds, and walnuts, only small amounts are converted to EPA and DHA. Eating 1–2 portions of fatty fish a week will ensure you reach your omega-3 targets. If you don't eat fish, a supplement containing EPA and DHA, derived from fish or algae, is recommended, in addition to including ALA-rich foods in your diet.

- **Iron** is an essential fertility and pregnancy nutrient (see p.67). Meat, fish, and eggs are all sources of iron, so if you don't include these in your diet, you need to ensure that you replace them with plant-based iron sources, such as pulses, tofu, nuts, seeds, green leafy vegetables, some dried fruit, and fortified foods. It's important to bear in mind that animal sources of iron are most easily absorbed by the body. Consuming sources of iron with food or beverages high in vitamin C enhances iron's absorption, so include foods or drinks with vitamin C (see p.64) alongside plant-based iron sources. Conversely, some polyphenols—plant-based compounds—in tea and coffee can inhibit iron's absorption, so it's best to avoid these drinks around mealtimes.

- **Vitamin B12** (see p.63) is a nutrient that's found naturally in animal products only, so if you follow a vegan diet, it's important to take a B12 supplement, or eat at least two servings a day of foods fortified with vitamin B12. Vegetarians can also be low in this vitamin, so again, fortified foods or supplements may be considered.

- **Iodine** is an important fertility nutrient (see p.69). Fish and dairy are key iodine sources, so if you don't eat these, you'll need to consider other sources. Some plant-based milk alternatives are fortified with iodine, but check the label as its fortification isn't standard. Seaweed can have very high levels of iodine, but excessive iodine can affect thyroid health, so eating too much seaweed isn't recommended (see p.69). If you don't consume fish or dairy, a supplement may be advisable.

- **Choline** is key for female reproductive health (see p.69). It's found in small quantities in some pulses and vegetables, but its richest sources are animal products such as meat and eggs. You may need to consider a supplement if your diet doesn't include these. Prenatal supplements often exclude choline, so additional supplementation may be needed.

Your key nutrients

Proteins, carbohydrates, and fats are macronutrients—the cornerstones of your diet that provide your body with energy and play a role in supporting your fertility.

Eat enough protein

Protein, a vital macronutrient, builds and repairs muscles and bones and is needed to make hormones and enzymes. It provides all the essential amino acids—the building blocks of protein that support egg and sperm development. Proteins are either complete—with all the essential amino acids; or incomplete—with low levels of, or missing, essential amino acids. Complete proteins tend to come from animal-based sources such as meat, fish, dairy, and eggs, and some plant foods such as soy, quinoa, and chia seeds. Incomplete proteins are mainly from plant-based sources such as pulses, nuts, and seeds. If you don't eat meat or dairy, including a range of plant-based proteins in your meals across the day will ensure you get all the essential amino acids.

If you eat animal-based foods, try to mix your protein sources. Research suggests that, compared to animal-based protein, plant-based protein is linked to a reduced risk of ovulatory infertility. Meat does supply important fertility-supporting nutrients, such as iron and vitamin B12, but processed and red meats in particular are associated with reduced sperm count. Both sexes should eat meat such as beef, lamb, and pork no more than three times a week. Women should consume 8–12 ounces of seafood per week, from choices lower in methylmercury (see p.31). For women undergoing fertility treatment, a high fish intake is associated with increased birth rates.

Protein is filling so a higher intake may be helpful if a fertility goal is to lose weight. A higher protein (more than 25 percent), lower carb (less than 40 percent) diet is also linked to increased pregnancy rates in IVF. Protein can also help manage PCOS (see p.18), which is often accompanied by insulin resistance (see p.19), as protein helps to stabilize blood sugar levels and regulate insulin.

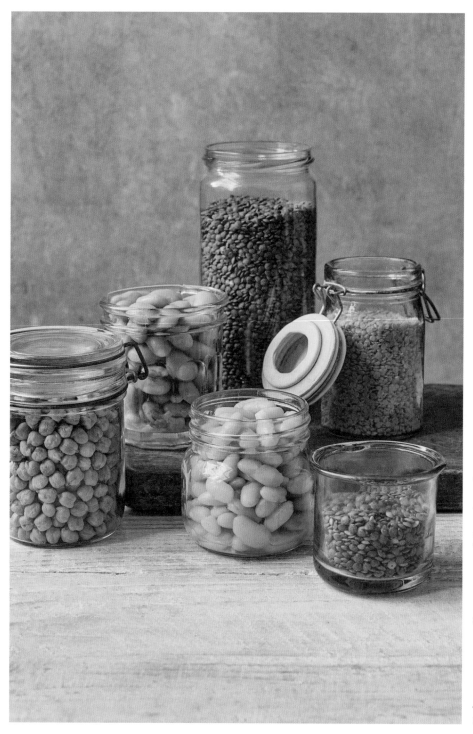

Pulses are an excellent source of plant-based proteins, as well as fiber and micronutrients.

The relationship between soy and fertility

Soy is a nutrient-dense and lean source of plant-based protein. It also contains all nine essential amino acids, which means it's a complete protein. Studies indicate that including soy in your diet can help promote many aspects of health, and it's thought that soy may play a protective role that can help reduce the risk of conditions such as cardiovascular disease and certain cancers.

Despite this, the relationship between soy and fertility remains a controversial one, so why does soy attract such attention? Soy is the main dietary source of isoflavones. Isoflavones are a type of antioxidant phytoestrogen—plant-based compounds that have a similar chemical structure to the estrogen our bodies produce. This means that isoflavones exert mild estrogenic effects on the body, leading to the suggestion that soy could have a negative effect on fertility by affecting hormonal balance. However, studies into the relationship between soy and fertility indicate that eating a low to moderate amount of soy a day—which could be one soy-based main meal or a drink—is not likely to be problematic, and may even help women with fertility issues. Occasional days with higher intakes are unlikely to cause a problem. In addition, soy is a good alternative to protein sources high in saturated fats, such as red meat, and an important protein source if you're following a plant-based diet— with the bonus that plant-based proteins are linked to a reduction in ovulatory issues. A study in 2020 on American and Danish women found that phytoestrogen intake wasn't associated with lower pregnancy rates, and some research suggests that, for women, eating soy when undergoing fertility treatment could improve the chance of a successful pregnancy and birth. For men, an analysis of 41 studies concluded that a moderate soy intake does not affect the reproductive hormones.

However, soy should not be eaten in excess because it's thought that a high intake could affect hormonal balance in women, in turn, impacting ovulation, and also sperm parameters in men. One study on men attending a fertility clinic showed that a high soy intake was associated with a lower sperm concentration, especially in men who were overweight or obese, although soy intake didn't appear to affect sperm count, motility, or morphology.

Is dairy helpful for fertility?

As well as being a rich source of protein, dairy is a principal source of calcium and contains other important fertility-promoting nutrients such as iodine and vitamin B12. Healthy eating guidelines recommend eating two to three portions of dairy a day. If you follow a plant-based diet with no dairy, you should opt for fortified plant-based alternatives that are enriched with at least calcium and iodine.

Fermented dairy products such as yogurt are also a source of probiotics—the good bacteria populating the gut. Your gut microbiome can influence your immune system, digestion, and potentially fertility. Gut imbalances can activate the immune system, triggering a chronic inflammatory response that can lead to insulin resistance, a common feature of PCOS (see p.18). Studies on the benefits for fertility of taking supplements of probiotics and prebiotics (compounds that feed good gut bacteria) show that in women with PCOS, this helped balance testosterone levels, reduced inflammation, and improved blood glucose levels and insulin resistance. Probiotics can also help maintain a healthy vaginal microbiome—the bacteria that live in your vagina—which may promote fertility and may support the endometrial microbiome, and in turn implantation.

Research also suggests that dairy supports levels of anti-müllerian hormone (AMH; see p.22), good levels of which point to a healthy ovarian reserve.

Despite these positives, dairy's impact on fertility has come under scrutiny. A key concern has been that its saturated fat content could cause inflammation (contributing to conditions such as PCOS). However, a review of 52 clinical trials found that neither high- nor low-fat or fermented dairy caused inflammation, and that, for reasons not fully understood, dairy could actually have an anti-inflammatory effect. In addition, the largest study to date looking at the links between dairy consumption and fertility in over 18,000 women showed that full-fat dairy was linked to a 50 percent reduced risk of ovulatory infertility, while low-fat milk was associated with an 11 percent increased risk. It is important to note that these findings have not been replicated. For men, though, lower-fat dairy may be preferable for fertility as it's associated with a higher sperm concentration and healthy motility.

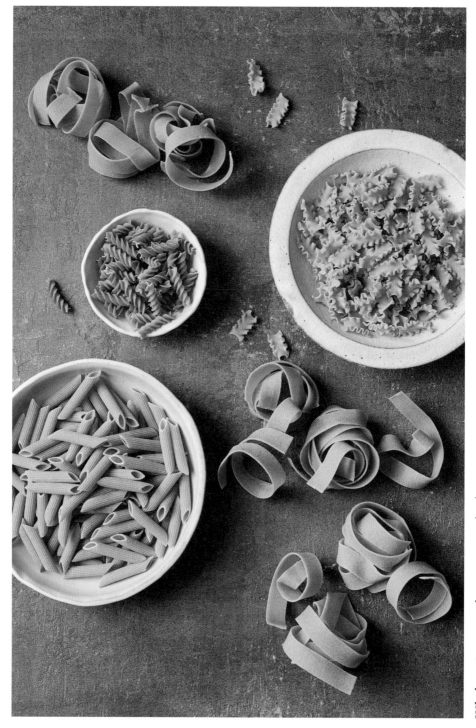

Whole grain pasta releases energy slowly, *helping to maintain healthy levels of insulin.*

Choose nutrient-dense carbohydrates

Carbohydrates are a key dietary source of energy. All of the complex processes involved in reproduction, such as hormone production, egg production and maturation, and sperm production require energy.

However, although carbohydrates play an important role in your diet, research suggests that ensuring that your intake isn't too high can help to lower insulin levels and balance hormones, in turn, helping to maintain regular ovulation, which can be especially beneficial for women with PCOS (see p.18). A moderate carbohydrate intake—with carbohydrates accounting for about 40 percent, or less, of your energy intake—could be a strategy to consider if you're trying to conceive.

Which carbohydrates should you eat?

Carbohydrates include starchy foods such as bread, pasta, and grains, and starchy vegetables such as potatoes. Sugars are also a form of carbohydrate, including natural sugars found in fruit and milk; and added sugars, commonly found in sugary drinks, sweets, cakes, and cookies. While carbohydrates can be a great source of fertility-supporting nutrients, it's important to consider both the quantity and the type of carbohydrate you eat and choose ones that are most nutrient-dense.

Whole grain carbohydrates contain zinc, folate, fiber, and a range of antioxidants, which are all supportive of fertility. As their name suggests, whole grains contain the entire grain—the bran (the fibrous outer layer with B vitamins and minerals); the germ (the nutritious inner core with healthy fats and vitamins); and the endosperm (the starchy middle section that includes protein and vitamins). This gives them a higher nutritional value than refined grains, which have been milled, removing both the bran and the germ—and with them important fertility-supporting nutrients. Some refined flours or breads are fortified with added vitamins after processing, but typically fiber isn't added back in.

Fiber is a key fertility nutrient. It's a type of carbohydrate, but it isn't broken down into glucose like other carbohydrates. Instead, it travels through the gut, where most of it is excreted undigested but some is fermented by gut bacteria. Research suggests that eating processed carbs rather than fiber-rich ones is linked to reduced pregnancy rates.

Good fiber sources include seeds, oats, brown rice, pulses, whole grain bread and pasta, potatoes and sweet potatoes with their skin on, and all other fruits and vegetables.

- Whole grains release energy more slowly than refined grains, helping to stabilize your blood sugar levels throughout the day and reduce the risk of insulin resistance, inflammation, and hormonal imbalances, all of which impact fertility. Insulin resistance is a key feature of PCOS (see p.18), so for women with this condition, switching from refined to whole grains lowers the diet's glycemic load (see pp.52–53) and can be particularly helpful.
- Eating more whole grains has been linked to healthy endometrial thickening, making the endometrium receptive to implantation.
- Ensuring that you consume more whole grains than refined carbohydrates is thought to help lower levels of inflammation in the body, in turn supporting fertility.
- A higher intake of whole grains in women has been linked to an increased chance of a successful cycle for couples undergoing IVF.
- A high fiber intake is associated with a reduced risk of experiencing ovulation-linked fertility problems. One study found that women who ate 1oz (25g) or more of fiber a day had a 13 percent higher chance of pregnancy than those who ate less than ½oz (16g) of fiber a day.

Does gluten affect fertility?

Gluten is a protein found in cereal grains such as wheat, rye, and barley, which means that it's present in many carbohydrate-rich foods such as pasta, bread, and cereals. There's some debate over whether gluten impacts fertility. Most people can process gluten, however, those with the autoimmune condition celiac disease are unable to tolerate gluten. If they eat gluten-containing foods, the body attacks itself and damages the gut lining, which in turn impairs the absorption of nutrients in the gut and causes a range of problematic symptoms. If you suffer with celiac disease, a strict gluten-free diet is essential to manage the condition.

Research suggests that having undiagnosed, or unmanaged, celiac disease may be an underlying cause of fertility problems in some women. This is thought to be caused by the condition leading to the malabsorption of nutrients. Left unmanaged, these can result in nutritional deficiencies that in turn can impact fertility. However, studies show that when women with celiac disease follow a strict gluten-free diet, they have no increased risk of fertility problems. Undiagnosed celiac disease can be a reason for unexplained fertility; therefore, if you have unexplained fertility, it's advisable to ask your health-care provider to screen you for celiac disease. If you're diagnosed with celiac disease, you can manage the condition with a gluten-free diet.

In some cases where celiac is ruled out, people report an intolerance to gluten that causes gastrointestinal symptoms, referred to as "non-celiac gluten sensitivity." However, there's no evidence that this affects fertility.

For women suffering with endometriosis—a painful condition where tissue similar to uterine tissue grows outside of the uterus—studies suggest that a long-term gluten-free diet could help to reduce pain in some people. This could make it easier for couples to enjoy sexual intercourse, in turn supporting the likelihood of becoming pregnant.

There are also anecdotal reports that a gluten-free diet could help to improve PCOS symptoms, although there's currently no evidence to support this. Furthermore, aside from the specific examples above, where gluten might negatively impact fertility, there's no evidence to suggest that cutting gluten out of your diet will have a beneficial effect on your fertility. In fact, because gluten is found in many fertility-supporting nutritious foods, eliminating gluten could potentially increase the risk of you not getting enough of some essential nutrients such as folate, iron, and fiber. Therefore, if you do decide to avoid gluten in your diet, it's important to discuss this first with a registered dietitian nutritionist, who can help you plan your diet carefully to ensure that you're not at risk of nutritional deficiencies that could impair both your health and fertility.

Blood sugar levels and fertility

Both the type and quantity of the carbohydrates you eat can influence fertility. Carbs are broken down into glucose—or sugar—which enters the bloodstream. This triggers the release of the hormone insulin, which promotes the uptake of glucose into your cells for energy. If insulin levels are too high, this can unbalance hormones and impact fertility.

Thinking about the glycemic index (GI) and glycemic load (GL)

A food's GI status (see opposite) describes the speed at which glucose is released from a carbohydrate-containing food. A food or meal with a high GI ranking means that sugars are released quickly into the body, leading to spikes in blood sugar levels and, in turn, raised insulin. In contrast, low GI foods release glucose slowly, allowing for a gentler insulin response.

If insulin levels are consistently raised, this can unbalance hormones, leading to higher levels of inflammation and increasing levels of damaging free radicals in the body. This, in turn, affects egg quality and processes such as implantation. Specifically, eating too many high GI foods, such as sugary, processed breakfast cereals, white rice, and some potatoes, has been associated with ovulatory problems, while a lower GI intake, including foods such as fruit, vegetables, whole grains, oats, chickpeas, and lentils, is associated with a reduction in ovulation-linked fertility issues. A low GI diet is also advised for women with PCOS (see p.18).

The glycemic load (GL) takes into consideration both a food's GI and the total amount of carbohydrate in a portion of that food, estimating how much blood glucose will rise following its consumption. Research suggests that a high GL diet also increases the risk of ovulatory problems in women as well as low sperm counts in men.

Avoiding a high-carb diet and making low GI swaps where possible will help you maintain a low GL diet. However, bear in mind that a food's GI ranking isn't the whole picture nutritionally. Pairing a carbohydrate with fat or protein lowers its GI, which means that high-fat foods such as chocolate can have a low GI. Likewise, some high GI foods can still be nutritious. A sensible approach, therefore, is to use GI as a guide but follow general healthy eating guidelines (see pp.38–41), as a food's overall nutrient profile may override its GI status in terms of nutritional value for fertility.

Breads

Rye 41

Oat bran bread 44

Mixed grain 52

White pita 57

Rye crispbread (seed crackers) 63

White bagel 69

White bread 70

French baguette 95

Pasta and rice

Brown rice, steamed 50

Instant noodles 52

White basmati rice 52

Wild rice 57

Linguine 61

Regular couscous 65

Gnocchi 68

Quick-cook white rice 87

Vegetables and fruit

Dried apricots 32

Apples 40

Strawberries 40

Bananas 47

White potatoes, boiled 54

Corn 55

Sweet potatoes, boiled 61

Dates 62

Raisins 64

Beets 64

White mashed potatoes 83

Grains, pulses, and nuts

Cashews 25

Kidney beans 29

Black beans 30

Chickpeas 36

Bulgur wheat 46

GI values of different foods

Lower GI foods have a gentler effect on blood glucose and, in turn, your body's insulin response, while higher GI foods produce a blood glucose spike. Generally, higher fiber, less processed foods have a lower GI, although there are exceptions.

Low GI = 0–55

Medium GI = 56–69

High GI = 70–100

The values here are taken from the University of Sydney GI database. Values from different sources may vary depending on factors such as brands and varieties.

Opt for healthy fats

As well as being a source of energy, fat plays an integral role in the production of hormones—a vital part of reproduction. You need small amounts of healthy fats in your diet to help your reproductive system work to its full potential. Fat is also needed for your body to absorb and use the fat-soluble vitamins A, D, E, and K.

Types of fat

Being aware of how different types of fat support your health and fertility can help you make the best choices. Focus on including sources of healthy mono- and polyunsaturated fats in your diet and limit saturated fats. Trans fats—a byproduct of a process called hydrogenation—found in some margarines and fast and processed foods, are consistently linked to poor health and fertility-related outcomes in both sexes so are best avoided.

- **Monounsaturated fats** have anti-inflammatory properties and are one of the main components of a Mediterranean-style diet. They're linked to a lower risk of cardiovascular disease and thought to improve pregnancy and birth rates. Olive oil, avocados, nuts, and seeds are good sources.

- **Polyunsaturated fats** include omega-3 (and omega-6) essential fatty acids. Omega-3s play a key role in a fertility-friendly diet and may be especially helpful for women over the age of 35. Two types of omega-3—docosahexaenoic acid (DHA) and eicosapentaenoic acid (EPA)—have key reproductive and anti-inflammatory benefits, supporting egg and embryo quality and implantation, and sperm quality. Fatty fish such as salmon, mackerel, and sardines are the best source of these omega-3s. Omega-3 alpha-linolenic acid (ALA) is found in flaxseeds, chia seeds, and walnuts, however, its conversion to EPA and DHA in the body is poor.

- **Saturated fat** is found in meat, dairy, and coconut oil. Foods containing saturated fat contain fertility-supporting nutrients. For example, meat supplies iron and vitamin B12; while dairy products such as yogurt have fertility benefits (see p.47). However, too much saturated fat can raise cholesterol levels and is linked to inflammation; research indicates a high intake can lower sperm count and concentration, so it's best to keep your total intake low and aim to consume more unsaturated than saturated fat.

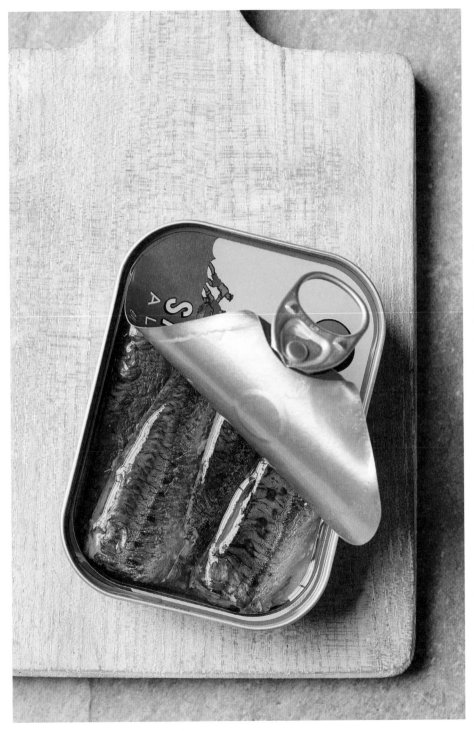

Fatty fish such as sardines are a rich source of omega-3 essential fats, a key fertility nutrient.

Increasing your fruit and vegetable intake

Fruits and vegetables are a rich source of protective antioxidants, a key part of a fertility diet. They also contain a whole range of vitamins and minerals—or micronutrients—many of which are also antioxidants. Fruits and vegetables are also low in calories, making them a useful tool for managing weight.

How much fruit and vegetables should I eat?

Healthy eating recommendations are to eat at least 14oz (400g) of fruit and vegetables (excluding potatoes) a day. A good practice is to divide this into five approximately 3oz (80g) portions of different fruits and vegetables. If you eat more than five servings a day, this can add to the fertility benefits. The diagram to the right illustrates what a portion of different types of fruits and vegetables can look like.

Fruit contains natural sugars, so if you are concerned about sugar, you could consider limiting your fruit to three portions a day. A glass of fruit juice counts as one of your five portions but should count for no more than this because of its sugar content. Fresh, frozen, canned, and dried fruit and vegetables all provide valuable nutrients. Pulses and beans also count as part of your "five a day."

It's best to rinse fruits and vegetables to reduce pesticide residue, which can impact pregnancy (see p.31). Although organic produce has fewer pesticides, it's still best to wash all fruit and vegetables thoroughly. It's also preferable nutritionally to leave edible peel on produce after washing as this is where fiber, nutrients, and antioxidants are often concentrated.

A good source of fertility-supporting antioxidants

While antioxidants are found in a variety of foods—including whole grains, herbs, plant-based oils, nuts, seeds, lean meat, seafood, and in tea and supplements— fruits and vegetables are an especially rich source.

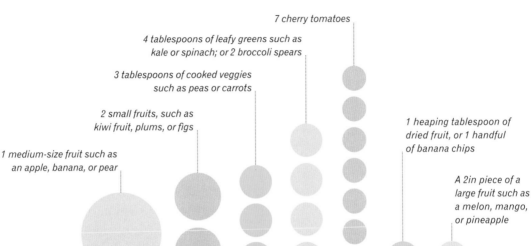

7 cherry tomatoes

4 tablespoons of leafy greens such as
kale or spinach; or 2 broccoli spears

3 tablespoons of cooked veggies
such as peas or carrots

2 small fruits, such as
kiwi fruit, plums, or figs

1 medium-size fruit such as
an apple, banana, or pear

1 heaping tablespoon of
dried fruit, or 1 handful
of banana chips

A 2in piece of a
large fruit such as
a melon, mango,
or pineapple

What does one "portion" look like?

There's considerable confusion around what makes up one portion of fruit or vegetable. This illustration shows how a portion can be a range of sizes and quantities depending on what you're eating.

An antioxidant-rich diet has clear fertility benefits. It's thought to improve egg and sperm quality, increase the chance of conception and a healthy pregnancy (including via fertility treatments), reduce conception times, and lower miscarriage risk. Antioxidants also improve sperm parameters, with studies correlating a low vegetable intake in men with a low sperm count. Antioxidant compounds can stop or slow the damage caused to cells by free radicals. High levels of free radicals and oxidative stress reduce the quality of eggs and sperm and affect fertilization and implantation rates as well as early embryo development. Increased levels of oxidative stress have been found in women with unexplained fertility problems.

An imbalance of free radicals and antioxidants increases oxidative stress. Antioxidants help neutralize free radicals by stopping them from causing damage. Not only do antioxidants protect us from the negative effects of free radicals, it's also thought that they can actually reverse some of the damage. Maintaining a balance between free radicals and antioxidants is therefore crucial for your well-being and reproductive health.

The natural phytochemicals that give fruit and vegetables their colors are often antioxidants, so eating a wide variety of produce can help you consume as many different antioxidants as possible. Key antioxidant nutrients that are abundant in fruits and vegetables include carotenoids as well as vitamin C, vitamin E, selenium, and zinc (see pp.64–67).

Carotenoids include the antioxidant compounds lycopene and beta-carotene. Lycopene, a potent antioxidant, is thought to be especially beneficial for sperm. Studies show that supplementing with lycopene can reduce sperm DNA damage and support sperm count, concentration, and morphology—or shape. Lycopene is found in some foods and drinks that have a red pigment, such as tomatoes (fresh and processed), tomato juice, watermelon, pink grapefruit, goji berries, pink guava, red cabbage, red peppers, and papaya. Beta-carotene converts to vitamin A in the body, which supports egg and embryo health. Beta-carotene is commonly found in brightly colored fruits and vegetables, such as apricots, butternut squash, and sweet potatoes.

Other benefits

Many types of fresh produce act as pre- or probiotics, promoting gut health and also benefiting fertility. As well as foods such as yogurt (see p.47), fermented vegetables such as kimchi, pickled vegetables, and sauerkraut act as probiotics, which may improve levels of healthy bacteria in the gut; while a wide range of fruits and vegetables, including onions, garlic, leeks, and unripe bananas, act as prebiotics, feeding the existing healthy bacteria. Optimizing your gut health is thought to support the balance of estrogen in your body.

Certain vegetables—such as beets and green leafy vegetables—contain dietary nitrates. These convert to nitric oxide in the body, which acts as a vasodilator, meaning it widens the blood vessels. This is thought to be beneficial for fertility as it can improve the blood flow to the uterus to support the chances of an embryo successfully implanting.

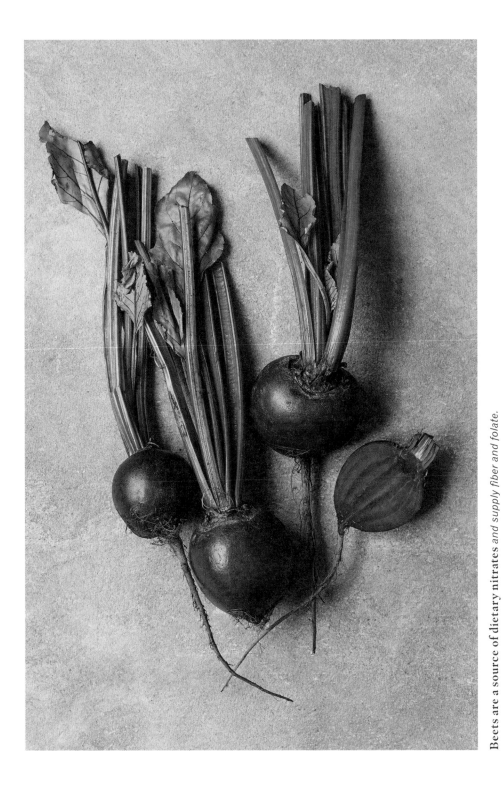

Beets are a source of dietary nitrates *and supply fiber and folate.*

Focus on micronutrients

A healthy, balanced diet provides a host of vitamins and minerals—essential micronutrients that help your body carry out many vital processes. For both women and men, ensuring that your diet provides good amounts of certain nutrients key to fertility enhances egg and sperm health and supports both natural and assisted conception.

Vitamin A

Also known as retinol, vitamin A supports the working of your immune system and plays a role in both male and female reproduction. In women, vitamin A is important for egg and embryo health and fetal development, while in men, a sufficient intake of vitamin A supports spermatogenesis—the production of sperm.

Foods such as fatty fish, eggs, and dairy products such as cheese, milk, and yogurt are all good sources of vitamin A, so incorporating these foods into your diet regularly will help to ensure that your body is getting adequate levels of this vitamin. You can also support your vitamin A levels by consuming good sources of beta-carotene, which is described as a pro-vitamin A carotenoid because it can be converted into retinol—or vitamin A—in the body. Sources of beta-carotene include spinach, kale, carrots, sweet potatoes, red peppers, red cabbage, mango, papaya, and apricots.

Liver is a particularly rich source of vitamin A. However, in pregnancy, high vitamin A levels aren't recommended because they can harm the developing fetus. Liver and liver products such as pâté should therefore be consumed with caution when you're trying to conceive and avoided if there's a possibility that you might be pregnant. Check supplements, too, to ensure that they don't contain high levels of vitamin A in the form of retinol. As well as avoiding high vitamin A food sources and supplements, the advice is to also avoid retinol-based skincare products in pregnancy.

The family of B vitamins

B vitamins are a class of water-soluble vitamins that play a range of important roles in the body, from facilitating energy production to supporting your nervous system and making red blood cells. Certain B vitamins also play essential roles in reproduction.

Vitamin B6

Also known as pyridoxine, vitamin B6 helps the body use and store energy from food and to form the substance hemoglobin, which is essential for carrying oxygen around the body in the blood.

Vitamin B6 is important for fertility as it's associated with healthy progesterone levels, so this means that it supports the luteal phase of your menstrual cycle (see p.11), when implantation could take place if an egg is fertilized. Avoiding a deficiency in this vitamin is thought to help reduce the risk of early pregnancy loss. Reliable sources of vitamin B6 can be found in foods such as poultry, fish, soy beans, oats, bananas, and peanuts.

Vitamin B9—folate

Folate, or vitamin B9, is the natural form of the prenatal supplement folic acid (see p.71) and it plays a major role in many aspects of fertility. Folate is important for the formation of DNA and healthy red blood cells and for the synthesis of amino acids, which in turn supports the development of follicles and other cells involved in reproduction, including endometrial cells. It has antioxidant properties and is important for supporting healthy ovulation, egg maturation, egg quality, progesterone production, and the successful implantation of an embryo. It also supports the development of the neural tube (the embryonic brain) in early pregnancy. Low levels of folate have been connected to an increased risk of miscarriage. For women, ensuring you have an adequate folate intake is one of the ways to enhance your fertility.

Folate is also a key nutrient when it comes to men and fertility. Research indicates that men who consume higher amounts of folate have a lower risk of having sperm with abnormal DNA.

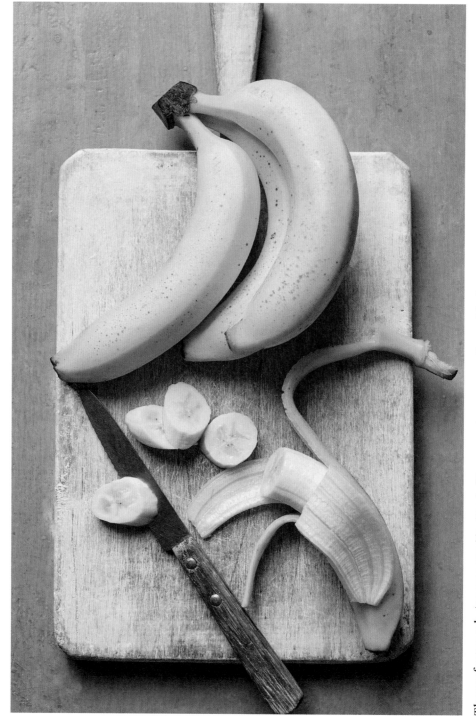

The perfect snack, *bananas provide vitamin B6, a progesterone-supporting nutrient.*

It isn't possible to consume sufficient vitamin B9 for your fertility and pregnancy needs through food sources alone, so all women who are trying to conceive are advised to take a 400mcg supplement of folic acid in the 12 weeks prior to conception and for the first 12 weeks of pregnancy, when the neural tube is forming. In addition to taking a supplement, incorporate folate-containing foods into your daily meals to sustain a healthy folate intake. Green vegetables are especially rich in folate, so include plenty in your diet—try green leafy vegetables such as kale, spinach, spring greens, and cabbage. Other dietary sources include asparagus, avocado, pulses, citrus fruits, edamame, mung bean sprouts, peas, lentils, beets, broccoli, feta, pears, pomegranates, corn, and fortified cereals and wheat bran. As a general guide, including two portions of green vegetables daily will help you to boost your folate intake.

Vitamin B12

Low levels of vitamin B12 are associated with both male and female fertility problems. Both folate and vitamin B12 are important regulators of the genes expressed in your DNA, known as DNA methylation, which plays a key role in the development of early life in the womb. If vitamin B12 levels are too low, this can lead to problems with ovulation. It can also reduce the ability of an embryo to implant in the uterus and it increases the risk of miscarriage. In men, a deficiency in vitamin B12 can lead to reduced sperm count, motility, and DNA damage.

Studies show that maintaining adequate levels of vitamin B12 improves implantation rates. One study even found that women who took a vitamin B12 supplement during fertility treatment had a higher chance of a successful cycle and pregnancy.

Vitamin B12 is found naturally only in animal products such as dairy, fish, shrimp, meat, eggs, and cheese. If you don't eat these foods regularly, consider taking a supplement or include two to three servings of foods fortified with vitamin B12 in your meals each day.

Vitamin C

This vitamin's antioxidant effects are thought to promote egg quality, ovulation, and progesterone levels, in turn aiding implantation and uterine health. A higher than normal intake is linked to shorter conception times in women with a BMI below 25. In men, vitamin C intake is linked to higher fertilization rates. It's believed to support several sperm parameters, including reduced DNA damage, as its antioxidant action protects sperm from oxidative damage. Vitamin C promotes iron absorption when paired with iron-containing foods. Oranges are often thought of as the top vitamin C source, but broccoli contains more. It's also found in other citrus fruits, kiwi fruit, apples, berries, apricots, peppers, Brussels sprouts, potatoes, and kale.

Vitamin D

As well as being important for bones, teeth, and muscles, vitamin D promotes reproductive health. A deficiency is linked to ovulatory problems, longer conception times, and a higher miscarriage risk. For women having fertility treatment, a successful cycle is more likely with sufficient vitamin D. Studies also show that vitamin D levels are significantly higher in men with good fertility, and there's strong evidence that it supports sperm motility. It's estimated that around 40 percent of pregnant women are vitamin D deficient. In warm weather, our skin synthesizes vitamin D from sun exposure, but in winter months it's hard to get enough vitamin D from food so a supplement is key (see p.72). Foods with small amounts include fatty fish, egg yolks, mushrooms exposed to UV light, and some fortified spreads and cereals.

Vitamin E

This is a potent antioxidant. In women, a deficiency is linked to fertility issues, and, in pregnancy, to increased miscarriage risk, early delivery, preeclampsia, and fetal growth problems. For women over 35, getting enough vitamin E is associated with shorter conception times, and its antioxidant effects are also thought to improve endometrial thickness and the womb's readiness to receive an embryo. For men, it protects sperm from oxidative damage. Research shows that taking vitamin E and C supplements together reduces sperm DNA damage. Food sources include avocado, vegetable oils, olives, apricots, nuts, and sunflower seeds.

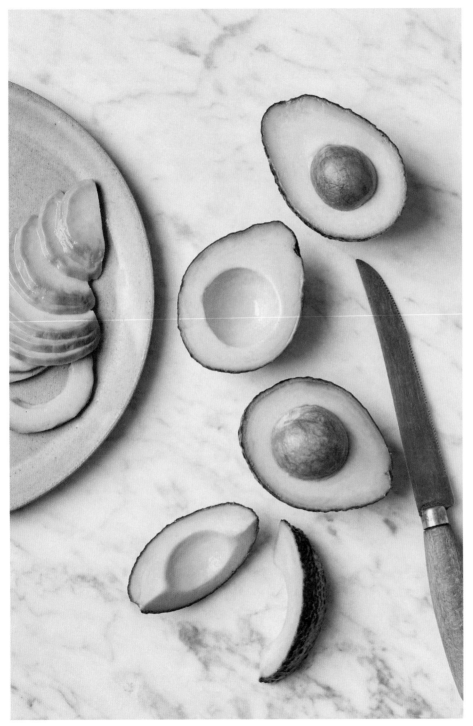
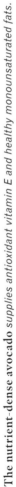

The nutrient-dense avocado supplies antioxidant vitamin E and healthy monounsaturated fats.

Selenium

Selenium is an essential trace mineral; we need just small amounts of it, but it's crucial for vital processes in your body. It plays a significant role in the reproductive health of both women and men—its powerful antioxidant action being key to its protective role in fertility. Where high levels are found in follicular fluid—the fluid surrounding the egg—it's thought that this enhances the quality of developing eggs. Conversely, if levels are low, this may negatively impact egg quality. Studies also indicate that low levels in women may prolong the time it takes to conceive.

Once pregnant, its antioxidant properties are thought to help sustain pregnancy by combating the effects of oxidative stress, and low levels in pregnancy are associated with an increased risk of miscarriage.

For men, selenium is needed for both sperm production and to protect sperm from oxidative stress. Adequate levels of selenium in men's diets support healthy sperm parameters such as motility—or movement.

Dietary sources of selenium include Brazil nuts, beef, pork, poultry, eggs, fish and seafood, oats, cottage cheese, mushrooms, and tofu. While it's key to ensure your body has this nutrient, an excess can have side effects, so it's best to ensure you don't get too much selenium. Brazil nuts are especially high in selenium, so limit your intake of these to no more than approximately two a day, which is generally sufficient to meet your quota.

Zinc

This mineral is also an essential trace element that plays a role in many important functions in your body. It acts as an antioxidant and is crucial for the regulation of cell growth, the release of hormones, the body's immune response, and reproduction.

Zinc is very important for male fertility. It helps to maintain normal levels of testosterone, and studies show that men who experience fertility problems have significantly lower levels of zinc in their seminal plasma—the fluid that carries sperm after ejaculation—compared with fertile men. Zinc may also support healthy sperm parameters (see p.14), such as volume, concentration, good sperm motility—or movement—and a good percentage of sperm having a normal morphology—shape and size.

For women, zinc plays an important role in the healthy maturing of eggs, as well as in ovulation, fertilization, and fetal development.

Zinc can be found in foods such as meat, poultry, eggs, dairy, shellfish, potatoes, leafy green vegetables, whole grains, kidney beans, chickpeas, almonds, cashews, oats, and pumpkin seeds. Bear in mind that zinc from animal sources is more easily absorbed by the body, so if your diet is plant-based, you need to incorporate sufficient amounts of zinc-rich plant-based foods into your diet to ensure that you're getting an adequate intake. You could also consider supporting your intake with a supplement.

Iron

Iron is an essential mineral that is crucial for oxygen transport and storage in the body, and it also helps support your immune system.

An iron deficiency, known as iron-deficiency anemia, is one of the most common nutritional deficiencies experienced by women. Iron is essential for reproductive health. It supports ovulation and is vital in pregnancy, where low levels are associated with an increased miscarriage risk, low birth weight, and premature birth. In women of childbearing age, iron needs are higher because iron is lost each month during the menstrual cycle. If you have heavy periods, you may be losing high amounts of iron each month, putting you at an even greater risk of a deficiency.

There are two types of dietary iron. Iron from animal sources, such as meat, poultry, and fish, is called heme iron, while iron from plant-based sources is called non-heme iron. Sources of non-heme iron include tofu, beans and pulses, quinoa, green leafy vegetables, sweet potatoes, nuts and seeds, dried fruits, oats, pasta, breads, and fortified cereals. Bodies absorb heme iron more easily than non-heme iron. However, research shows that an iron intake from iron supplements or from non-heme iron sources is associated with a reduced risk of ovulatory infertility, which suggests that plant-based sources of iron in particular could play a significant role in female fertility.

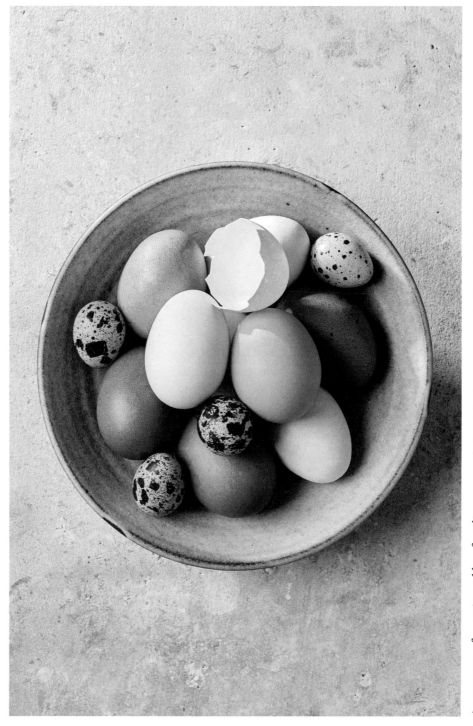

As a source of protein and key fertility-supporting nutrients, *eggs are a valuable part of a fertility diet.*

Choline

This is described as a brain-building nutrient. An adequate intake of this nutrient during pregnancy is linked to a healthy placenta and good fetal neural development—it may even impact cognitive function into childhood. It's also thought to help protect against the development of certain birth defects such as neural tube defects.

Sources of choline include beef, eggs, chicken, salmon, pork, milk, Brussels sprouts, cauliflower, broccoli, legumes, mushrooms, and nuts. Animal sources usually contain a greater concentration. Because this nutrient isn't included regularly in prenatal supplements, diets and supplement plans—in particular for those following a plant-based diet—should be carefully tailored to ensure they contain sources of choline.

Iodine

This essential nutrient influences many aspects of health and plays an especially important role in thyroid health. Low iodine levels have been linked to taking a longer time to conceive. Iodine is essential for the synthesis and release of thyroid hormones, which are involved in ovulation, so maintaining sufficient levels supports normal ovulation. Adequate iodine levels also support optimal pregnancy outcomes, while severe deficiencies have been linked to an increased risk of pregnancy loss. Women's iodine status in pregnancy has also been linked to fetal brain development, which may even impact school performance.

Iodine deficiency isn't uncommon, especially in young women and pregnant women, so it's important to ensure you're getting enough of this vital nutrient. Milk, other dairy, fish, and shellfish are its main sources. Eggs, meat, nuts, bread, and some fruits and vegetables also have iodine, but in lower amounts. Seaweed contains iodine, but this can be in very high amounts. Regular consumption of seaweed isn't advised because there's a risk of iodine "toxicity," which can affect thyroid health. Kelp supplements also aren't advised for this reason. If your diet is low in dairy—especially milk—and fish, you may be deficient in iodine, so consider talking to your health-care provider about taking a supplement.

The role of supplements

Vitamins and minerals (see pp.60–69) play a crucial role in many reproductive processes, supporting egg maturation, egg and sperm quality, and implantation, as well as protecting against oxidative stress. Improving your micronutrient status is therefore one way you can enhance your fertility. Prioritizing and optimizing your diet is key and shouldn't be neglected. For many women, though, a prenatal supplement supports nutrient intake when trying to conceive. Supplements may have fertility benefits for men, too.

When are supplements helpful?

Most prenatal supplements are made up of a combination of the many essential vitamins and minerals involved in reproduction. Not only do they include essential nutrients that women are advised to supplement before and during pregnancy—such as folic acid—but they can also fill in nutrient gaps in your diet, minimizing the risk of deficiencies that could impact fertility. This can be especially helpful if you omit certain food groups, for example, if you follow a vegan or vegetarian diet. By restoring a healthy micronutrient status, supplements can benefit both women without known fertility issues and those struggling to conceive, as their antioxidant action helps to combat oxidative stress, helping to reduce conception times and increase the chance of pregnancy. Evidence suggests that, alongside diet, women who take a regular prenatal supplement have a reduced risk of fertility problems related to ovulation.

Some prenatal supplements are targeted at men. These contain antioxidant nutrients designed to lower oxidative stress levels and support sperm quality. Research suggests that taking antioxidant supplements is generally beneficial for male fertility.

The following is a selection of supplements that can support fertility. Some may be included in a prenatal supplement; otherwise, you may wish to supplement separately. If you take multiple supplements, make sure you're not getting an excess of any nutrient. Some have safe upper limits, so don't exceed this amount without medical approval. When navigating fertility supplements, it's wise to seek support from a doctor ore registered dietitian nutritionist specializing in fertility.

Folic acid/methylated folate

Folic acid is the synthetic form of folate (vitamin B9, see p.61) in supplement form. It's a crucial nutrient for helping to reduce the risk of neural tube defects developing in early pregnancy. It's not possible to get all of the folate you need to reduce this risk from dietary sources alone. Therefore, women are advised to take 400mcg folic acid while trying to conceive, 600mcg during pregnancy, and 500mcg while breastfeeding.

Sometimes a higher folic acid dose is advised, which a doctor needs to prescribe. Situations when this may apply include if:

- *a previous pregnancy was affected by a neural tube defect, or you have a family history of neural tube defects.*
- *you have diabetes.*
- *you're very overweight (see pp.24–25).*
- *you have sickle cell disease.*
- *you're taking certain epilepsy medications.*
- *you take antiretroviral medicines for HIV.*

Some prenatal supplements contain a different type of folate, known as 5-methyltetrahydrofolate (5-MTHF), or methyl folate. This is aimed at a minority of women who have the genetic variation MTHFR C677T, which affects how the body metabolizes folic acid. Some experts believe that the efficacy of folic acid has limitations in women with this mutation who have experienced failed IVF, recurrent miscarriages, and/or stillbirth. As a result, they suggest that where this genetic mutation is found, women can benefit from taking a supplement with methylated folate. However, there's a lack of evidence supporting this advice. The main concern of recommending methyl folate is that there isn't research to prove its effectiveness in preventing neural tube defects, and for ethical reasons, it's unlikely that this research will take place. However, there has been no data to suggest that methyl folate is harmful, and the UK Teratology Information Service, commissioned by Public Health England, has said that methyl folate could be considered in cases where its benefits are likely to outweigh the risks to the mother or baby. Understanding this discussion can help you to make an informed decision, with the support of your health-care provider, about which type of folate supplement to take if you know you have this genetic variant.

Folic acid's, or methylated folate's, antioxidant action means that it's also included in some supplements for men.

Vitamin D

This vitamin promotes reproductive health in men and women (see p.64), supporting sperm health, ovulation, conception times, and IVF. It's hard to get enough vitamin D from diet alone. Your body synthesize it from sunlight so a supplement is especially helpful in the winter months. For fertility, a daily supplement of 10mcg is advised, at least in the winter months, taken on its own or as part of an prenatal supplement. If you are deficient in vitamin D, you may need a higher dose to achieve sufficient levels. You should consult your doctor before making this decision, who can check your levels with a blood test and make a recommendation.

Coenzyme Q10

This antioxidant vitamin-like compound occurs naturally in the body. It plays a role in energy production and in fertility, providing energy for the enzymatic processes that are needed for egg production and embryo development. High levels in follicular fluid are linked to optimal embryo development and higher pregnancy rates. We get some coenzyme Q10 from food, but in research, benefits have been shown from a high-dose supplement. As we age, coenzyme Q10 levels naturally decrease. For women in their mid- to late-thirties onwards, seen as an advanced maternal age, a supplement supports egg and embryo quality. In men, it may improve sperm concentration, count, motility, morphology, and DNA fragmentation. Coenzyme Q10 supplements are found in two forms: ubiquinol or ubiquinone. Ubiquinol is more easily absorbed so considered more effective.

Omega-3 essential fatty acids

For women whose dietary omega-3 is low, an omega-3 supplement can increase the probability of conception when trying to conceive naturally. For men struggling to conceive, an omega-3 supplement may help to improve sperm parameters such as motility, count, concentration, and morphology. For men with a reduced sperm concentration in particular, an omega-3 supplement may be the most beneficial. If you don't eat one to two portions of fatty fish each week, an omega-3 supplement with both EPA and DHA (see p.54) will be beneficial and will ensure you're receiving adequate amounts.

Vitamin E

Supplementing this vitamin can be useful for women where embryos have failed to implant in IVF treatments. For men, it's thought that antioxidant supplements containing vitamin E might improve IVF outcomes where there's sperm DNA damage.

Inositol

Inositols are vitamin-like, naturally occurring compounds found in fiber-rich foods such as pulses, beans, whole grains, and fruit, nuts, seeds, meat, and eggs, but their benefits are more apparent in supplement dosages. The most common type of supplement is called myo-inositol; d-chiro inositol is another type. Studies show that a myo-inositol supplement may increase the pregnancy rate in women who are undergoing ovulation stimulation for IVF or intracytoplasmic sperm injection (ICSI). It's thought that supplementation may reduce the amount of unsuitable eggs and improve the quality of embryos and also reduce the amount of drugs needed to stimulate the ovaries.

For women with PCOS (see p.18), research has shown that myo-inositol, in combination with the prescribed medication metformin (a medication that's prescribed for use in PCOS to help manage insulin resistance), is associated with a higher live birth rate than when taking metformin alone. Other research suggests that myo-inositol alone can help normalize ovarian function and improve egg and embryo quality in women with PCOS. Some studies have also looked at whether myo-inositol or d-chiro inositol alone, or a combination of these, is most effective for PCOS and suggest that a combination of myo-inositol with a low dose of d-chiro inositol in a 40:1 ratio may be best for restoring ovulation in women with PCOS. If you're considering an inositol supplement, discuss these options with your health-care provider.

For men, a myo-inositol supplement can support sperm motility and mitochondrial function in sperm.

Probiotics

Research suggests probiotics can help balance the vaginal microbiome, an imbalance of which is linked to female fertility issues. Also, a low colonization of lactobacillus in the endometrium microbiome is linked to problems with implantation failure and pregnancy loss. Evidence also suggests that probiotics or synbiotics (a mixture of probiotics and prebiotics) may improve testosterone levels, decrease inflammation, and improve insulin resistance and blood glucose levels in women with PCOS, in turn improving fertility in these women. Much more research needs to be done in this area, but taking a probiotic with a lactobacillus strain may help to support fertility outcomes for some people—in addition to eating plenty of fruit, vegetables, nuts, seeds, and whole grains to promote a healthy gut microbiome.

Your fertility lifestyle

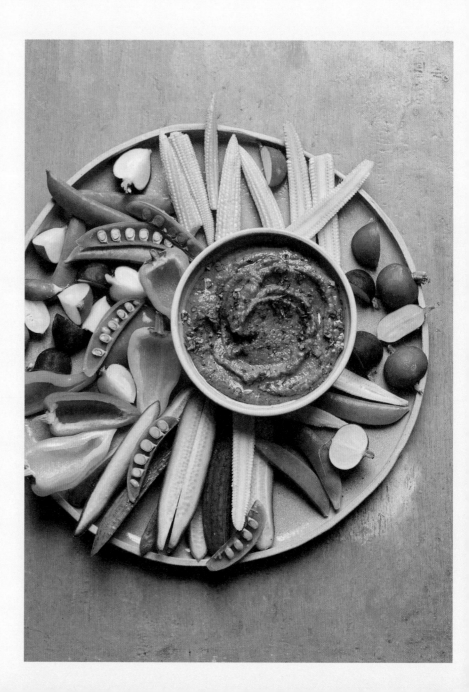

Alongside an optimal fertility diet, taking a whole lifestyle approach to supporting your health and well-being can positively influence fertility. How active you are, how soundly you sleep, and how you manage stress are all significant parts of the fertility puzzle. What's more, all of these areas are interconnected, so when you successfully manage one, it has a knock-on effect, improving other parts of your life.

The following chapter explains how these lifestyle factors can support both women's and men's fertility, helping to regulate hormones and support the body's natural processes. Guidance is offered on how to weave exercise and activity into your daily routine—and how to tailor exercise regimes to suit particular fertility circumstances. Helpful suggestions pinpoint ways to improve your sleep hygiene, with tried-and-true tips for getting to sleep and staying asleep.

Importantly, your response to stress can impact fertility— and for couples who are struggling to conceive, the path to pregnancy can be a source of stress in itself. Exercise and sleep are proven ways to help manage stress. Here, therapies and practices are also suggested that can help you cope with stress and support your path to conception and pregnancy.

Activity and exercise

As well as being good for general health, staying active can impact our fertility. For both sexes, a lack of activity can be detrimental to fertility outcomes—whether trying to conceive naturally or via assisted fertility treatments—and is associated with unexplained infertility (see p.16). In some situations, though, overexercising isn't advised. Being aware of the guidelines for your circumstances can help you shape your exercise regime to enhance your fertility.

How exercise can impact women's fertility

Getting the balance right between engaging in exercise and activity and overdoing it is very important for women's fertility. Being active before and during early pregnancy can reduce the risk of pregnancy problems. Public health guidance is to aim for a benchmark of 150 minutes moderate exercise or 75 minutes vigorous exercise a week, as well as strength and resistance work (see opposite). Studies show that more than 60 minutes vigorous exercise a day can increase the risk of anovulation (see p.19). If exercise causes your BMI to fall below 19 (see p.25), this may imbalance hormones and, in turn, impact ovulation and fertility. Conversely, doing between 30 and 60 minutes of vigorous activity daily—more than the benchmark—was thought to reduce this risk and support healthy ovulation.

For women with PCOS (see p.18), studies show that more vigorous aerobic exercise and resistance training (see opposite) can improve insulin sensitivity and lower high levels of androgens (male hormones).

Exercise and men's fertility

Generally, opting for the recommended 150 minutes of moderate activity or 75 minutes vigorous activity a week is thought to support men's fertility, while a lack of exercise can reduce testosterone levels, leading to a reduced sex drive and erectile dysfunction. Some research also shows that excessive exercise may affect male fertility by increasing oxidative stress and chronic inflammation in the body. This may, in turn, lower testosterone production and affect sperm parameters.

Building activity into your day

While integrating an exercise regime into your week has well-known benefits for fertility and general health, there are also benefits from simply increasing your daily activity, especially if you struggle to fit in or maintain a structured exercise routine. Building walks into your day, taking regular desk breaks, doing physical housework, gardening, or enjoying a dance all help to keep you active to support fertility.

How exercise can affect fertility

Men and women aged 19–64 are advised to get a certain amount of exercise each week. However, there are some caveats to this advice that may help enhance fertility in particular circumstances.

*If exercise has brought your **BMI below 19**, this can affect ovulation. Exercise should be reduced to no more than 150 minutes moderate exercise, such as walking or yoga, a week.*

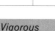

Moderate activity

*Getting at least **150 minutes** of **moderate aerobic activity** or **75 minutes** of **vigorous aerobic activity each week** (or a mix of these), plus 2 sessions of strength or resistance training, is the standard advice for all adults aged 19–64.*

Vigorous activity

Moderate aerobic activity includes brisk walking, moderate speed cycling, heavy housework, lawn mowing, swimming, dancing, and doubles tennis.

Vigorous aerobic activity includes jogging, fast cycling, singles tennis, soccer, and aerobics.

*If you suffer with **PCOS**, doing at least 120 minutes of vigorous exercise a week—more than the general recommendation—can be beneficial.*

***The risk of anovulation** is thought to be reduced by doing 30–60 minutes of vigorous exercise a day, but doing more than this can lead to ovulation problems.*

A sleep routine for fertility

Getting enough good-quality sleep is vital for our bodies and minds to function well. When trying to conceive, adequate sleep helps you cope with anxiety, provides the rest your body needs, and may also play a role in balancing hormones.

The link between sleep and fertility

It's thought that a lack of sleep, or experiencing disturbed sleep, for example, waking in the night, may be associated with reduced fertility. Hormones such as estrogens, progesterone, and androgens such as testosterone are regulated by your circadian body clock. So when you get insufficient sleep, this may affect the production of these important sex hormones. There's also a link between a lack of sleep and an increased risk of metabolic disorders, diabetes, depression, and obesity, all of which can impact fertility.

One of the key hormones that helps regulate sleep is melatonin, which is produced by the body after the onset of darkness and peaks in the middle of the night. Melatonin also acts as an antioxidant and has been associated with improved pregnancy rates in couples with unexplained infertility (see p.16) who are undergoing fertility treatment. The levels of melatonin the body produces naturally declines with age. Supporting your sleep can help to increase levels of melatonin naturally.

How much sleep do I need?

To maintain your mental and physical health, you should aim to get seven to nine hours of sleep each night. Regularly getting less sleep than this—for example, getting less than five to six hours sleep a night—can interfere with menstrual cycles and sperm parameters and affect both natural conception and IVF outcomes. Practicing good sleep hygiene—ensuring your environment and lifestyle support a healthy

Avoid smoking as nicotine is a stimulant.

Don't drink alcohol or eat too close to bedtime.

Create a calming bedtime routine.

Ensure that the room you sleep in is dark and cool.

Reduce the amount of caffeine you drink and limit, or ideally avoid, caffeine close to bedtime.

Avoid vigorous exercise in the evenings.

Switch off all blue light-emitting devices an hour before sleep.

Developing good habits for sound sleep

Integrating the sleep recommendations above can help you establish a healthy sleep routine to support fertility.

amount of sleep—will help you manage stress, enhance your physical health, and promote successful fertility outcomes.

- What you eat and drink and when can impact your sleep. Both caffeine and nicotine are stimulants. Giving up smoking enhances general health and fertility as well as your sleep. Some experts recommend avoiding caffeine-containing drinks after 12pm to ensure they don't disrupt your sleep. Drinking alcohol in the evening can also affect your sleep and eating food late in the evening can make it harder to fall asleep as your body is working to digest your food.

- While gentle exercise in the evenings may have no effect on sleep, vigorous exercise that raises your body temperature may make it harder to settle, so it's best to avoid strenuous exercise 1–2 hours before bedtime.

- Winding down before sleep is important to help you switch off. Find ways to relax, whether reading or taking a warm bath, to help you feel sleepy. Avoid looking at devices for at least an hour before bedtime, and make sure that your room isn't too hot and is sufficiently dark.

Managing stress

Advice often offered to couples trying to conceive is to "just relax and it will happen." If you and your partner have been struggling to become pregnant, this may not feel very helpful. However, it's thought that stress can sometimes have an impact on fertility, so finding ways to manage it can be an important part of your fertility journey.

How stress can affect fertility

The relationship between stress and fertility is actually quite complex and not one that we fully understand. Studies show that there is an association between stress and fertility, but it's not fully understood which is the cause and which is the effect.

Being on a fertility journey or struggling to conceive can be a very stressful experience. Women who are experiencing fertility problems have been found to have higher levels of stress than fertile women. This in turn leads to raised levels of prolactin—which can affect ovulation, higher levels of cortisol (the stress hormone), and increased anxiety. These physiological and psychological effects can impact conception outcomes, whether trying to conceive naturally or through assisted fertility techniques. Conversely, research also shows that women undergoing assisted fertility treatments who have lower levels of depression and anxiety are more likely to become pregnant. Stress can also have a negative influence on the quality of sperm.

Finding tools to reduce stress

Research shows that psychosocial interventions, such as cognitive behavioral therapy (CBT), counseling, and relaxation training, can improve psychological symptoms, such as anxiety, and lead to a significant increase in pregnancy rates among couples struggling to conceive.

While reducing your levels of stress may not be the whole solution to helping you conceive—especially if you know that you or your partner has a physical problem that is affecting fertility—it can help you to deal with problems that are associated with infertility, such as anxiety or discomfort caused by a physical concern, and support your overall well-being while you're trying to conceive.

There are a range of different practices that you can incorporate into your daily life to help you reduce your stress levels. The key is to prioritize stress-relieving activities—making them as important as other activities in your daily routine, such as going to work or cooking dinner.

Bear in mind that what works for one person may not be helpful for another individual. Finding an activity or practice that you enjoy and that works for you is therefore very important in ensuring that you create a lasting habit that will be most effective in enhancing your well-being. The following stress-relieving activities are all recommended.

- Try practicing mindfulness and meditation and/or incorporate breathing exercises into your daily routine.
- Join a yoga or Pilates class, where relaxation and breathing can form an important part of the practice.
- Consider acupuncture, which research suggests may help to reduce stress levels.
- Keep a gratitude journal, to help you focus on all of the positive elements in your life.
- Take time each day to do something you enjoy, whether that's exercise, relaxing in a bath, or reading a book.
- Talk to friends and family to build your support network.
- Take time out to enjoy a vacation or a short break.
- Spend time with your partner where you both consciously avoid thinking about trying to conceive.

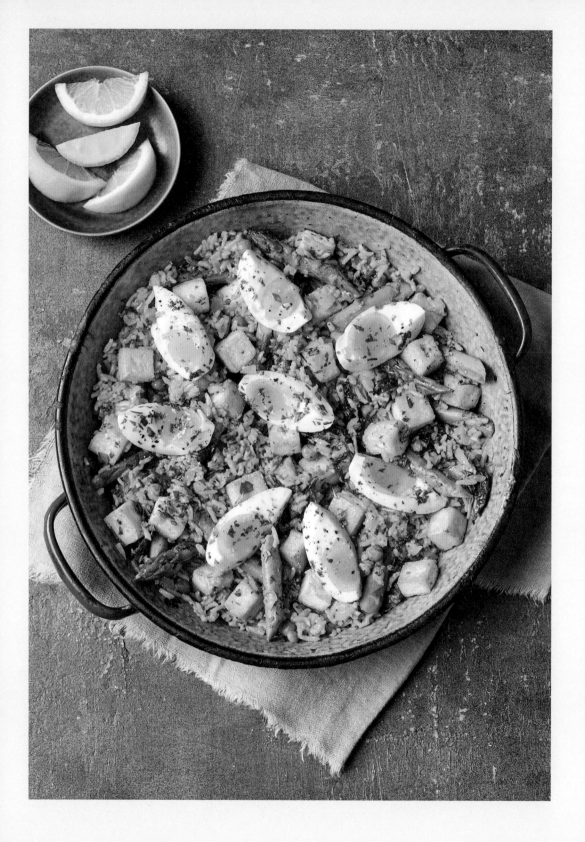

Recipes
for fertility

The following selection of more than 60 recipes provides delicious fertility-friendly ideas for each meal throughout the day, as well as a selection of nourishing beverages. Enjoy supporting your fertility daily with these nutritious and appetizing recipes.

Navigating the recipes

The recipes in the following section are designed to provide fertility-friendly, nutritious, balanced meals, healthy snacks, and beverages. Here are a few helpful suggestions for tailoring recipes, as well as some points on the ingredients and methods.

Tailoring your fertility diet

The recipes in this book can support the fertility of both women and men. The following suggestions can also act as a guide if you wish to focus on recipes that support a particular fertility situation or area.

- **Recipes with plant-based proteins** are thought to be especially supportive of healthy ovulation (see p.44). If regular ovulation and menstruation is a concern, as well as seeking professional advice and guidance, you may wish to make sure to include recipes with plant-based proteins such as pulses, beans, and tofu.
- **Consuming high-fiber** carbohydrates is associated with a higher chance of pregnancy. Choosing recipes with high-fiber carbs, such as breakfasts with oats and fruit and meals with pulses and beans and an abundance of vegetables, will help ensure a good intake of fiber.
- **Certain nutrients are key in early pregnancy.** Folate-containing ingredients such as leafy greens, beets, pulses, and avocado, are supportive of early pregnancy, as well as general fertility. Recipes with choline, found in ingredients such as eggs; iodine, found in eggs and in fish and dairy; and vitamins B6, C, and E in particular are also key in pregnancy. Include meals with these nutrients to support implantation.
- **Tomato-based meals** are an excellent source of lycopene, which supports healthy sperm parameters. Meals with zinc, found in seafood such as prawns, are also beneficial for sperm health.
- **Foods containing omega-3** may be especially helpful for egg

health—particularly in women in their mid- to late-thirties onwards, which is generally referred to as an advanced maternal age—and can help to optimize sperm quality. Choose recipes with fatty fish, such as salmon, mackerel, and sardines, as well as walnuts and chia, hemp, and flaxseeds. Remember to eat fatty fish no more than twice a week (see p.28).

- **Antioxidant-rich foods** may help protect egg and sperm cells from oxidative damage. Regularly include recipes that have plenty of vegetables, fruit, nuts, seeds, whole grains, and vegetable oils, especially extra-virgin olive oil.
- **For men** whose sperm concentration is known to be low, you may want to avoid eating large amounts of soy-based foods, such as tofu and edamame.

A few specifics

Some of the following recipes provide options for certain ingredients or specify a preference for a certain type of container for an ingredient.

- **For recipes with milk**, there are options for plant-based or dairy milk. Evidence suggests that high-fat dairy could support ovulation and low-fat dairy may support sperm health. These findings haven't been validated, but you may wish to follow these guidelines based on existing evidence. However, try not to worry too much if you consume the same milk as your partner. If using plant-based milk, choose one that's fortified with fertility nutrients such as calcium and iodine.
- **Throughout, whole wheat options** for bread, pasta, and grains are given (see p.26 and p.41) as these are best for fertility. However, if you find wheat difficult to tolerate, swap these for wheat-free alternatives.
- **The ingredient lists** suggest buying certain ingredients in cartons instead of cans. This is because cans can contain endocrine-disrupting chemicals (EDCs; see pp.30–31). Not everyone may wish to focus on reducing EDCs, but if you've experienced fertility issues, you may wish to limit your exposure. However, if an ingredient is hard to source in a carton, purchasing a can is okay. It's impossible to eradicate our exposure to all EDCs, but minimizing exposure where possible can be helpful.
- **Throughout the recipes**, convection oven temperatures are used. If you are using a standard oven, add 25 degrees to Fahrenheit temperatures.

Breakfasts

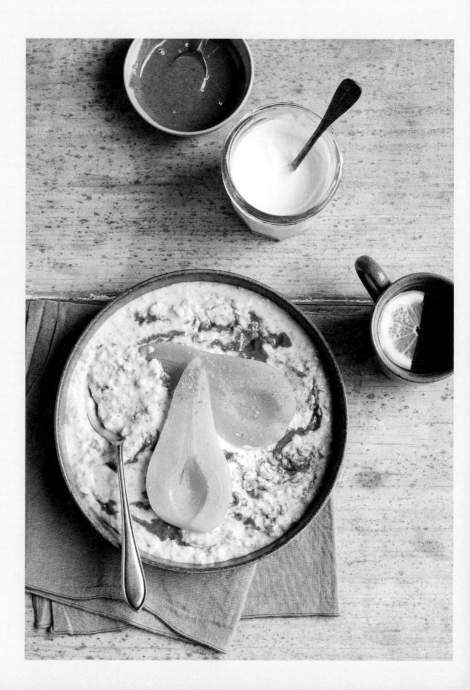

For many people, breakfast is often overlooked—sometimes skipped entirely or else a rushed affair with little thought given to its nutritional value and a reliance on sugary cereals.

This appetizing collection of quick-to-make recipes encourages you to rethink this first meal of the day and make breakfast count. Delicious sweet and savory options with antioxidant-rich ingredients and sources of fiber invite you to treat breakfast as an opportunity to replenish nutrients, refuel for the day ahead—and avoid those midmorning hunger pangs that can see you reaching for sugary snacks.

Enjoy creamy oats with summer berries or juicy pear; egg treats, such as kale and feta omelet or savory muffins; or whole wheat toast with nutrient-dense toppings. For busy mornings—or if you find eating first thing a struggle—whip up a nutritious smoothie. Flexes suggest quick swaps for vegan breakfasts, catering to a variety of dietary preferences.

Making a nutritious breakfast part of your daily routine is a valuable contribution to your fertility diet.

Chia, carrot, *and* pecan oats

provides antioxidants • aids egg and sperm quality • may support implantation

Chia seeds and flaxseeds are high in antioxidants and provide plant-based essential omega-3s, promoting egg and sperm health, while whole grains such as oats support implantation. Together, oats, seeds, carrots, and pecans create a low GI breakfast, steadying blood sugars, insulin, and other hormones.

Serves 1
Prep 5 mins
Rest 1 hour

1 tbsp chia seeds
¼ cup (30g) rolled oats
4¼fl oz (125ml) milk or plant-based alternative
½ tsp vanilla extract

pinch of ground cinnamon
1 tbsp (10g) raisins
½ carrot (about 1oz/30g), grated
1 tbsp Greek yogurt
small handful of pecans, crumbled
1 tbsp ground flaxseed

Place the chia seeds, oats, milk, vanilla extract, cinnamon, raisins, and carrot in a small bowl, container, or jar and mix together until evenly combined. Let stand for 1 hour.

Add the yogurt and stir once again, then top with the pecans and flaxseed. Enjoy right away, or keep the oats covered in the fridge for up to 3 days.

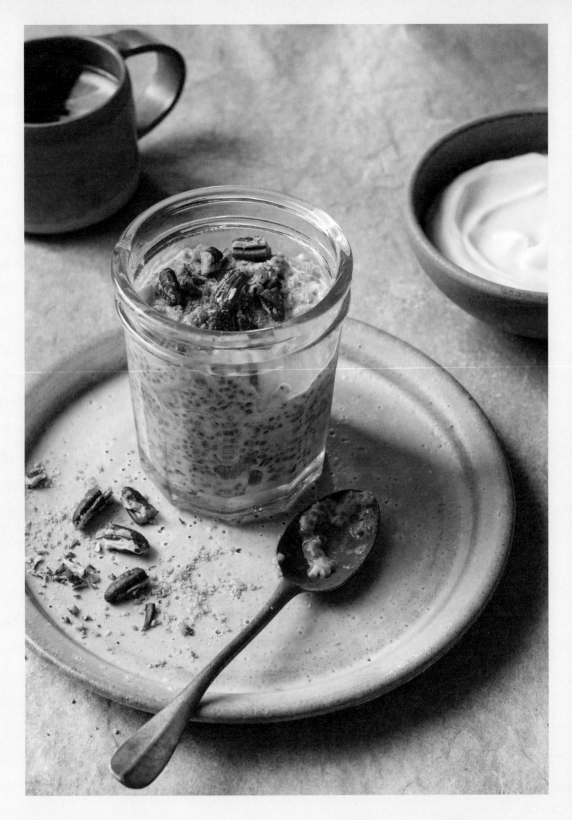

Chia, carrot, and pecan oats

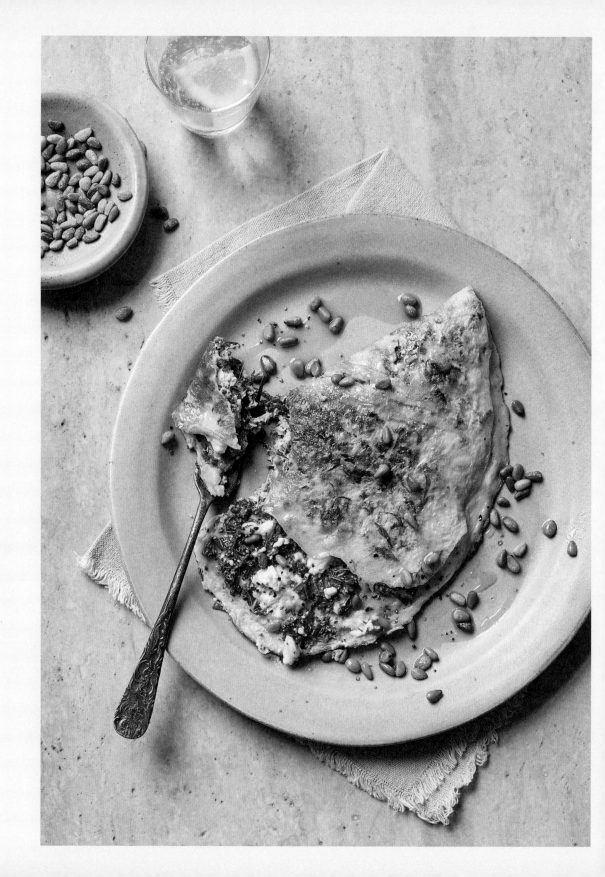

Kale *and* feta omelet

aids sperm health • provides antioxidants • supports early fetal development

This satisfying breakfast or brunch is nutritionally dense. Eggs supply protein; sperm-supporting zinc; and choline, key for early fetal development. Kale delivers a bundle of fertility-promoting antioxidants, including folate and vitamin C.

Serves 1
Prep 5 mins
Cook 5 mins

2 eggs
1 tbsp cottage cheese

handful of kale, finely chopped (or pulsed in a food processor)
1 tsp olive oil, plus extra to drizzle (optional)
2 tbsp (30g) feta, crumbled
1 tsp pine nuts

Whisk the eggs in a bowl, then use a fork to stir in the cottage cheese. Add the kale and stir to combine a little.

Heat the oil in a lidded skillet over medium heat. Once hot, pour in the egg mixture and swirl it to coat the base of the pan. Cook for about 2 minutes, until the eggs have just set. Place the feta on top and gently fold the omelet over. Cover and cook for another minute, until the filling is warmed.

In the meantime, toast the pine nuts for 2–3 minutes, stirring constantly, until golden. Serve the omelet while hot, with the pine nuts sprinkled on top and drizzle olive oil over the nuts if desired.

Watermelon *and* strawberry smoothie

Serves 2
Prep 5 mins

14fl oz (400ml) milk or
   plant-based alternative
2 tbsp Greek yogurt
²/₃ cup (100g) watermelon
   (fresh or frozen), diced
²/₃ cup (100g) strawberries
   (fresh or frozen)
ice, to serve (optional)

Selection of toppings
½ kiwi, sliced
1 tbsp pumpkin seeds
1 tbsp coconut flakes
handful of fresh mint
   leaves, chopped

Flex it—*For a vegan smoothie, opt
for plant-based milk and choose soy
yogurt for its protein content.*

**hydrates • aids sperm health • aids passage
of sperm**

This summery smoothie is a refreshing start to the
day. Watermelon's high water content hydrates,
helping optimize cervical mucus to aid the passage
of sperm; while its lycopene content supports
sperm concentration and morphology—or shape.

Place the ingredients for the smoothie in a blender
and pulse to a smooth consistency.

Pour the smoothies into 2 glasses, adding ice
if desired, and top with the preferred toppings.
Enjoy right away.

Avocado, pear, *and* lime smoothie

Serves 2
Prep 5 mins

½ **avocado**
1 **pear, peeled and cored**
juice of ½ lime
2 tbsp **Greek yogurt**
1 tbsp **rolled oats**
14fl oz (400ml) **milk or**
   plant-based alternative
ice, to serve (optional)

Flex it—*To make this a vegan
smoothie, opt for plant-based
milk and use soy yogurt for its
protein content.*

supplies fiber and folate • provides antioxidants

Creamy and with a hint of sweetness, this delicious smoothie includes low GI fiber-rich oats. Avocado and pear add folate, key for reproductive health, as well as antioxidant vitamins C and E.

Place all the ingredients in a blender and pulse to a smooth consistency.

Pour the smoothies into 2 glasses, adding ice if desired, and enjoy right away.

Beet burst smoothie

Serves 2
Prep 5 mins

1 beet, peeled and chopped
½ avocado
1 banana
handful of spinach
³/₄ cup (100g) mixed berries
   (fresh or frozen)
1 tbsp chia seeds
14fl oz (400ml) milk or
   plant-based alternative
2 tbsp Greek yogurt
ice, to serve (optional)

Flex it—*For a vegan smoothie,
opt for plant-based milk and choose
soy yogurt for its protein content.*

**aids egg and sperm quality • provides
antioxidants • may support implantation**

This irresistible smoothie packs in the goodness.
Beet has folate, for egg and sperm health, and
nitrates, which promote healthy blood flow to the
uterus. Avocado adds anti-inflammatory fats and
this colorful drink delivers a host of antioxidants.

Place all the ingredients in a blender and blend
to a smooth consistency. Pour the smoothie into
2 glasses, add ice if desired, and enjoy right away.

Scrambled eggs *with* garlic mushrooms *and* asparagus

Serves 1
Prep 5 mins
Cook 10 mins

1½ tbsp vegetable oil
handful of mushrooms
    (shiitake, button, or
    oyster), sliced
5 asparagus spears,
    tough ends chopped off
1 garlic clove, finely
    chopped
pinch of salt and freshly
    ground black pepper
2 eggs
1 tbsp milk or plant-based
    alternative
1–2 slices of whole wheat
    sourdough bread
1 tsp olive-based spread
handful of chives, sliced,
    to garnish

aids egg and sperm health • supports early pregnancy • supplies folate

This savory breakfast treat supplies selenium from the eggs and mushrooms, supporting egg and sperm health. Asparagus adds folate, important for egg and sperm health and a key nutrient for early fetal development.

Heat 1 tablespoon of the oil in a frying pan over high heat. Once hot, add the mushrooms and fry for 5 minutes. Reduce the heat slightly and add the asparagus spears and garlic. Season and cook for 2 minutes, stirring regularly, until the asparagus is softened.

While the mushrooms and asparagus are cooking, heat the remaining oil in a small saucepan over medium heat. Whisk the eggs in a small bowl and mix in the milk using a fork. Add the whisked eggs to the saucepan, season, and cook, stirring frequently, for 2–3 minutes, until they form soft curds and are cooked to your liking.

Toast the bread as preferred and then spread over a thin layer of the olive-based spread. Spoon the scrambled eggs onto the toast and top with the asparagus and mushrooms. Enjoy right away, garnished with the chives.

(photographed overleaf)

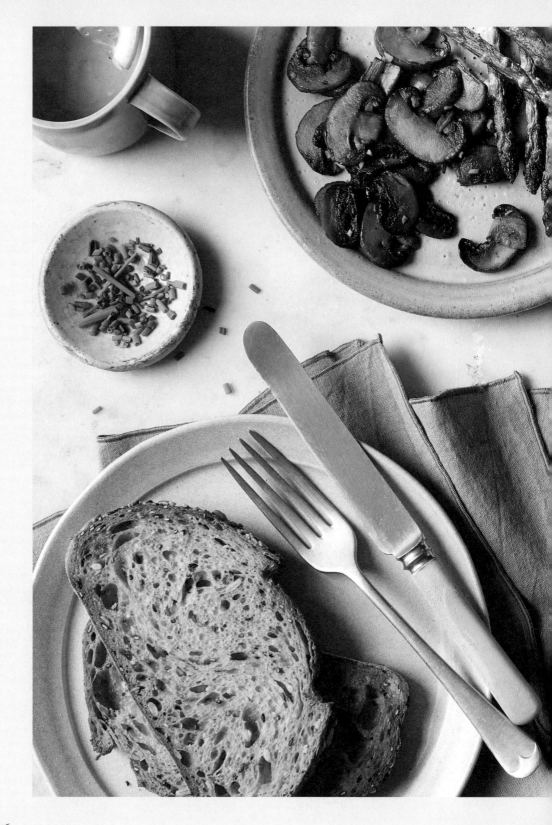

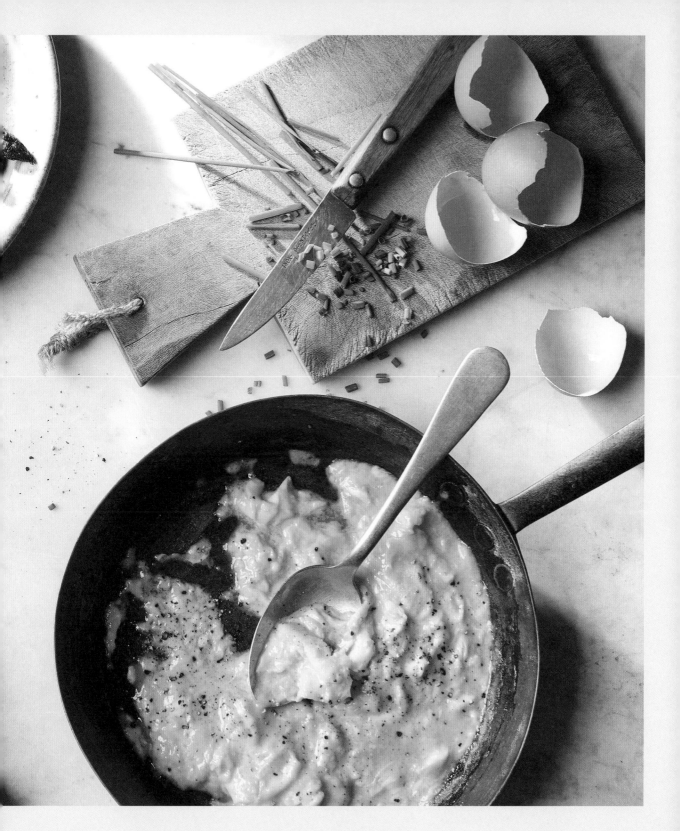

Scrambled eggs with garlic mushrooms and asparagus

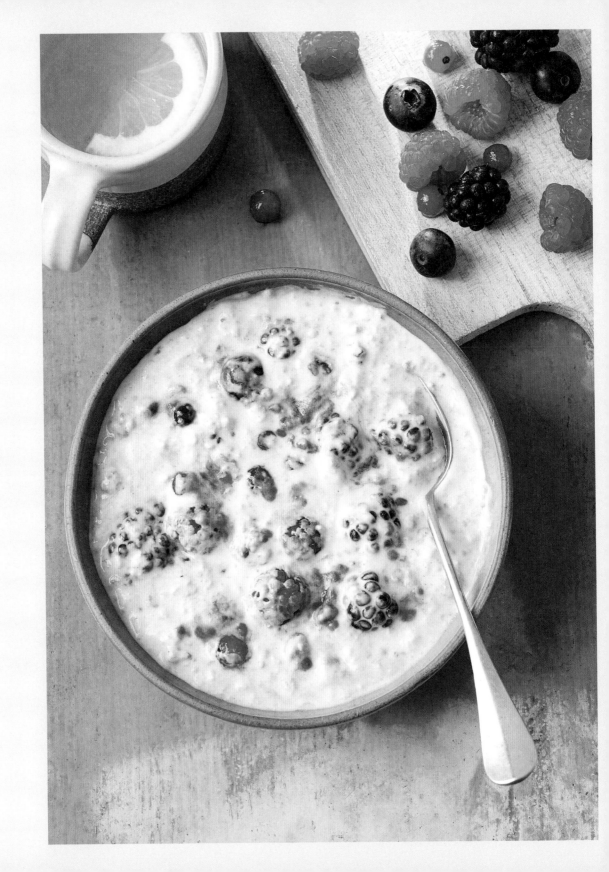

Berries galore overnight oats

supplies fiber • provides antioxidants

Creamy oats and sweet and refreshing berries make this breakfast bowl a winner. Whole grain oats supply fiber and key fertility nutrients such as selenium, zinc, and iron. Berries and chia seeds add a whole package of fertility-supporting antioxidants.

Serves 1
Prep 1 hour, or overnight

$^1/_2$ **cup (40g) rolled oats**
$^1/_2$ **cup (125g) natural yogurt**
5fl oz (150ml) milk or
 plant-based alternative
1 tsp chia seeds
$^3/_4$ **cup (100g) mixed berries,**
 fresh or frozen

Place the oats, yogurt, milk, and chia seeds in a bowl. Stir for a few minutes to prevent the chia seeds from clumping together.

Add the berries and mix all the ingredients together well. Cover and refrigerate overnight, or for at least an hour. Enjoy right away or store in an airtight container in the fridge for up to 3 days.

Flex it—*For an easy vegan swap, opt for a plant-based milk and choose soy yogurt for its protein content.*

Poached pear oatmeal

Serves 1
Prep 5 mins
Cook 15 mins

1 pear, peeled, halved
    lengthwise, and cored
1/2 tsp vanilla extract
1/2 cup (40g) rolled oats
7fl oz (200ml) milk or
    plant-based alternative
1/4 tsp ground cinnamon
1 tsp unsalted almond butter
1 tbsp natural yogurt
1 tbsp ground flaxseeds

Flex it—*For a vegan oatmeal,
opt for a plant-based milk and
choose soy yogurt for its
protein content.*

**aids egg and sperm health • may help reduce
conception time • has anti-inflammatory
properties • may support implantation**

Juicy and sweet, fiber-rich pears are a good source
of vitamin C, which is thought to promote shorter
conception times. Flaxseeds add anti-inflammatory
omega-3s and whole grain oats support implantation.

Bring a small lidded saucepan of water to a boil.
Once boiling, reduce to a simmer and add the pear
and vanilla extract. Cover and poach the pear for
15 minutes.

In the meantime, make the oatmeal. Place the oats,
milk, and cinnamon in a saucepan over medium heat.
Cook for 10 minutes, stirring frequently, until the
oatmeal is a creamy consistency.

Serve the oatmeal topped with the almond butter,
yogurt, flaxseeds, and the poached pear.

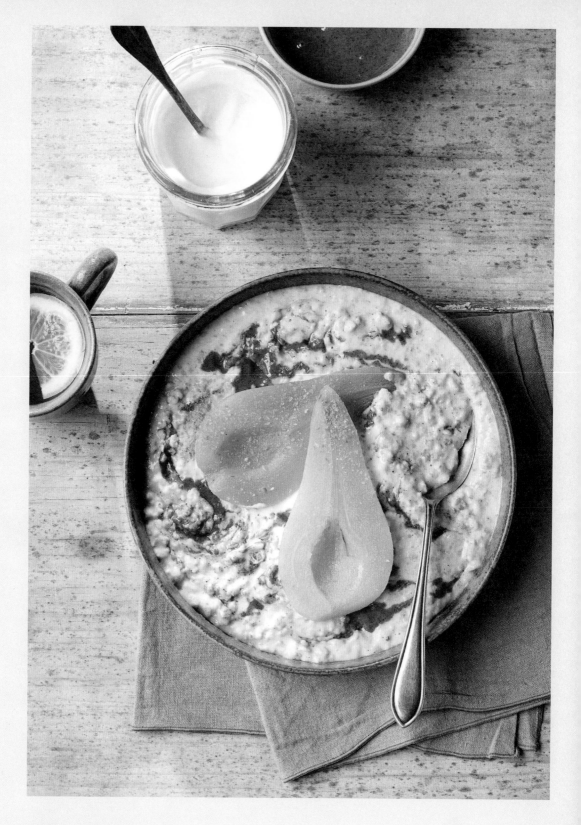

Poached pear oatmeal

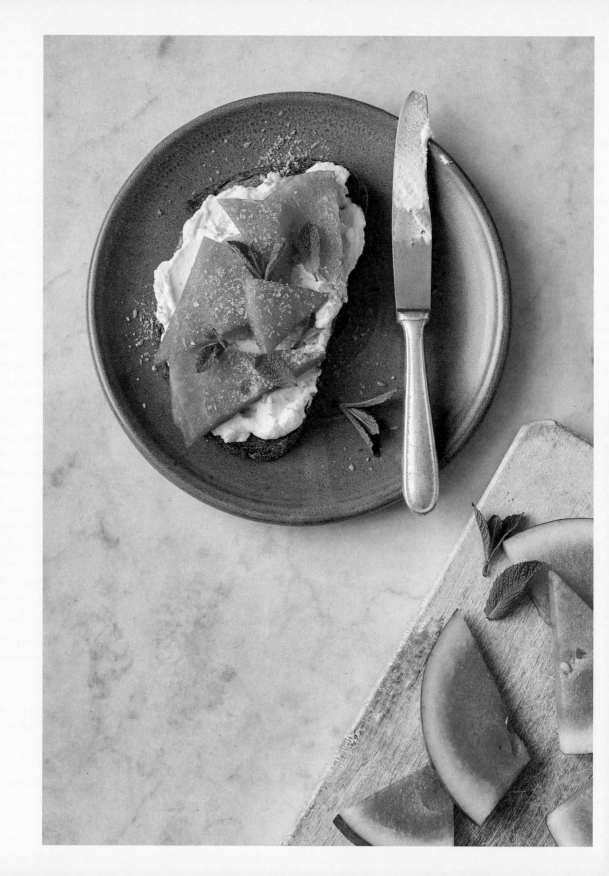

Watermelon *and* ricotta toast

aids passage of sperm • hydrates • aids sperm quality

Pep up your morning toast with this delicious ingredient combo. Creamy ricotta supplies essential protein, while refreshing watermelon helps hydrate the body—promoting healthy cervical mucus to facilitate the passage of sperm—and also supplies lycopene, promoting sperm quality.

Serves 1
Prep 5 mins
Cook 5 mins

1 slice of whole wheat bread
1–2 tbsp ricotta
$^1/_2$ tsp vanilla extract

$^1/_2$ cup (80g) watermelon, cut into 1in (2.5cm) pieces
1 tbsp ground flaxseeds, to garnish
mint sprigs, to garnish

Lightly toast the bread. Place the ricotta and vanilla extract in a small bowl and mix together, then spread this over the toast.

Top the toast and ricotta with the watermelon and garnish with the flaxseeds and mint.

Egg, feta, *and* zucchini muffins

Serves 1–2
Prep 5 mins
Cook 25 mins

1 tbsp olive oil
1 scallion, finely sliced
1 garlic clove, crushed
¼ zucchini, grated and
  excess liquid squeezed out
pinch of salt and freshly
  ground black pepper
2 eggs
1 tbsp milk or plant-based
  alternative
2 tbsp peas, fresh or frozen
4 cubes of feta

provides antioxidants • aids egg and sperm health • supports early fetal development

Hard to resist, these egg breakfast bites provide high-quality protein and antioxidants. Feta is a good source of folate and, together with eggs, vitamin B12, both of which are key for sperm health and important nutrients in early pregnancy.

Heat the oven to 425°F (200°C) and grease 2 of the cups in a muffin pan. Heat the oil in a skillet over medium heat and fry the scallion for 2 minutes. Add the garlic and cook for 1 minute. Add the zucchini, season, and cook for another minute, then set aside to cool.

Whisk the eggs and milk in a small bowl, using a fork, then add the cooled zucchini mixture and peas and stir to combine.

Divide the muffin mixture between the 2 greased muffin cups. Arrange the feta pieces on top of each cup. Bake in the oven for 15–20 minutes, until the eggs have puffed up and the center jiggles slightly when moved. Enjoy warm or cold.

If batch cooking, place in an airtight container and refrigerate for up to 3 days or freeze for up to 3 months.

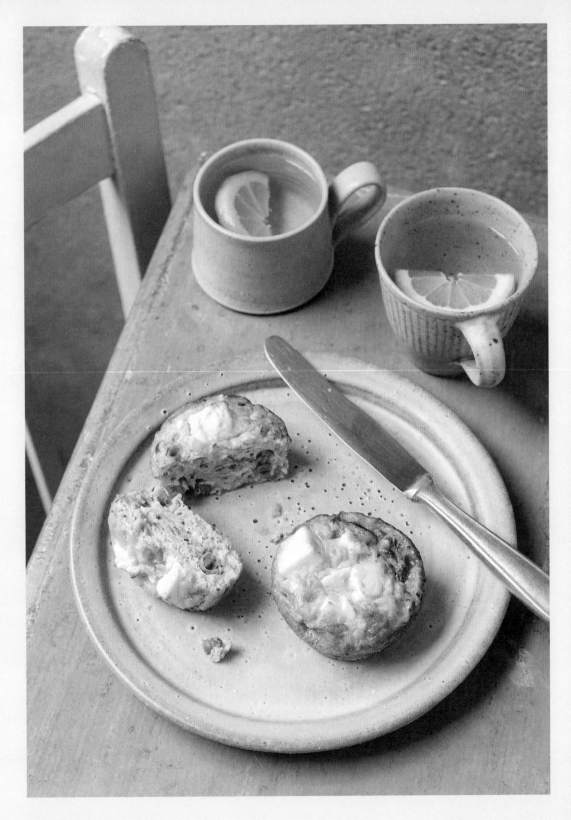

Egg, feta, and zucchini muffins

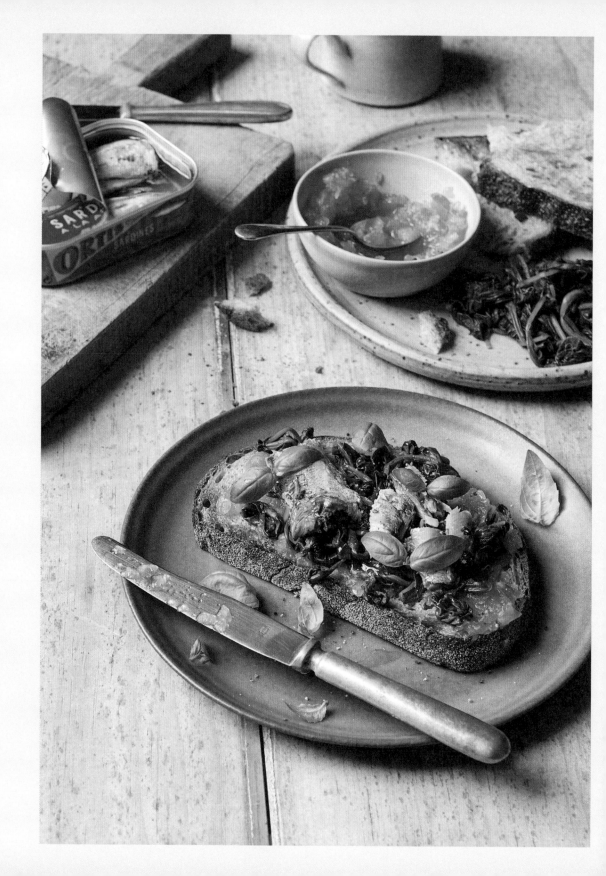

Breakfasts

Toast *with* tomatoes *and* sardines

Serves 1
Prep 5 mins
Cook 5 mins

**1 large beefsteak tomato,
   halved**
**pinch of freshly ground
   black pepper**
a large handful of spinach
**1–2 slices of whole wheat
   sourdough bread**
1 garlic clove, skin removed
1 tbsp extra-virgin olive oil
**4oz (120g) can sardines in
   spring water or olive oil
   (about 3oz/90g drained
   weight), flaked**
handful of basil leaves

**aids egg and sperm health • has
anti-inflammatory properties**

This traditional Spanish breakfast supplies the compound lycopene—in the tomatoes—thought to support a healthy sperm concentration and sperm shape. Sardines add anti-inflammatory omega-3s to promote both egg and sperm health.

Loosely grate the tomato into a bowl and season with pepper. Gently wilt the spinach over a saucepan of boiling water.

Lightly toast the bread. Rub the garlic clove over one side of the toast while the toast is still hot—to spread the garlic flavor—then drizzle over the olive oil. Spread the grated tomato over the toast and top with the wilted spinach and the sardines. Sprinkle on the basil and enjoy right away.

Light bites
and main dishes

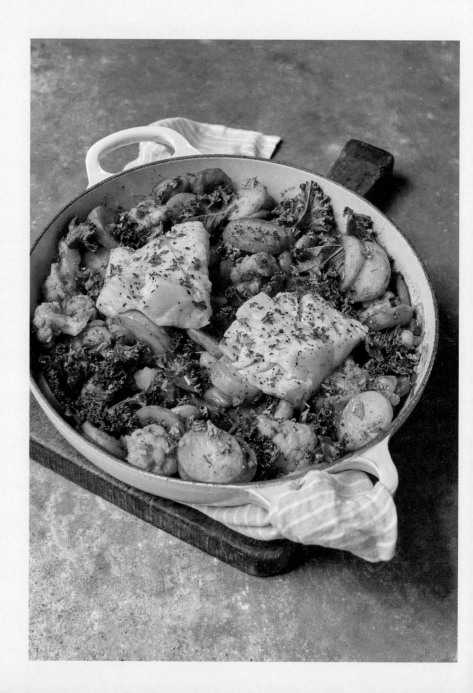

Your meals throughout the day need to provide sufficient energy to enable you to get on with everyday routines and supply a variety of nutrients to help your body function at its best. A fertility-supporting diet focuses in particular on meals with a low glycemic load, ensuring that energy is released slowly, which in turn keeps blood sugar levels—and hormones—stable.

The following chapter offers an appetizing selection of nutrient-dense meals. Lighter bites and dishes are great for quick lunches and dinners on busy days, while more substantial recipes are perfect for leisurely meals and weekend fare. All the recipes provide a balanced plate, full of valuable fertility-enhancing nutrients.

Choose from a mouthwatering selection of satisfying salads and pulse- or grain-based meals; try nourishing soup, enticing toast toppings, or a quick-to-assemble wrap; or enjoy a range of traditional favorites. Vegan, vegetarian, and meat-including diets are all considered—with flex ideas throughout for removing or adding meat and/or dairy while still delivering key fertility nutrients.

Bean salad bowl

Serves 2
Prep 5–10 mins

13.4oz (380g) carton cannellini beans, drained and rinsed
¼ red onion, thinly sliced
¼ cucumber, diced
½ orange pepper, seeded and diced
10 black olives, pitted and halved
12 cherry tomatoes, halved
1 avocado, peeled, pitted, and sliced
2 large handfuls of salad leaves or spinach
2oz (60g) mozzarella, torn into small pieces

For the dressing
1 tbsp extra-virgin olive oil
½ tsp Dijon mustard
½ tsp balsamic vinegar
handful of flat-leaf parsley, leaves only, chopped
½ tsp lemon juice
1 tsp mixed seeds

supports ovulatory health • supplies fiber • provides antioxidants

This satisfying salad is full of fertility-supporting nutrients. Plant-based proteins—from cannellini beans here—are linked to healthy ovulation. The veggie and bean medley is abundant in fiber and key antioxidants, including vitamin E from the avocado.

Place the beans, red onion, cucumber, orange pepper, olives, tomatoes, avocado, salad leaves or spinach, and mozzarella in a large bowl and toss to combine.

To make the dressing, place all the ingredients in a separate bowl and mix together with a fork. Pour the dressing over the salad and toss to combine. Enjoy!

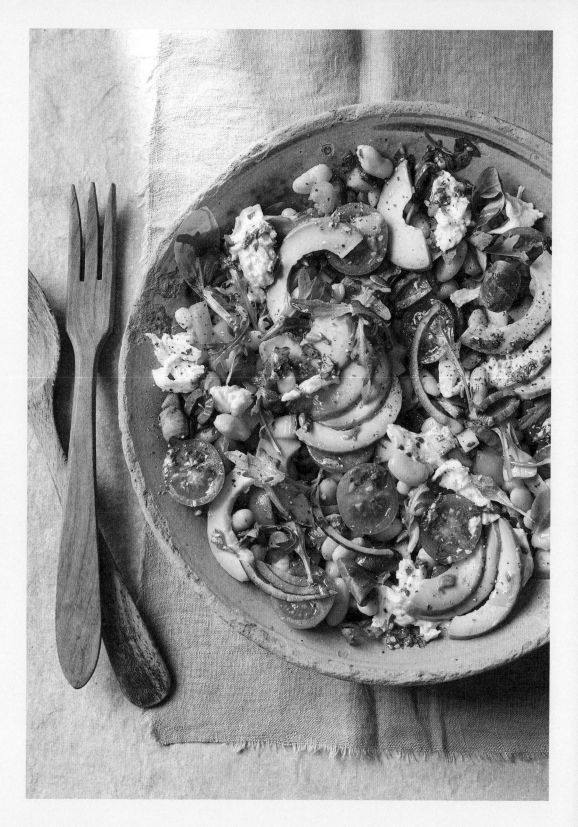

Bean salad bowl

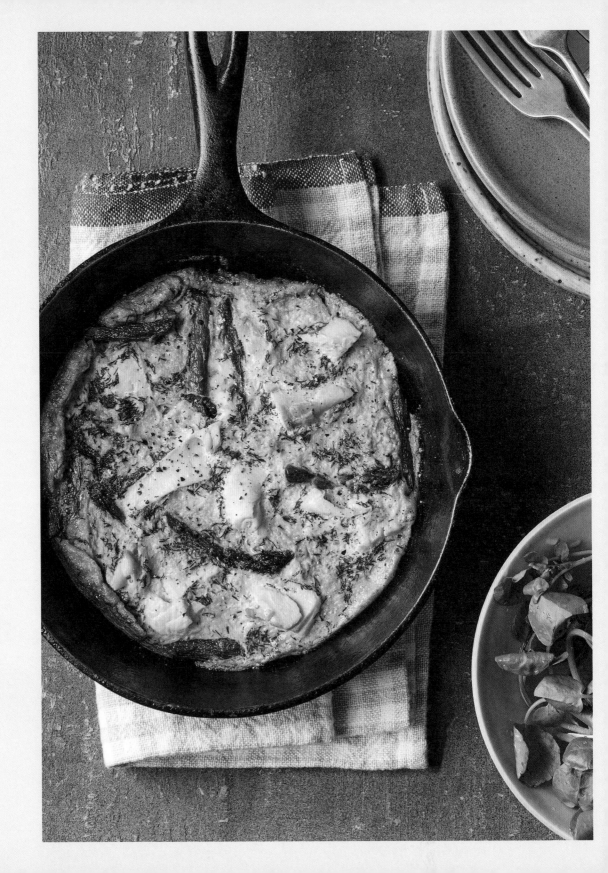

Salmon *and* asparagus frittata

Serves 2

Prep 5 mins

Cook 15 mins

1 tbsp olive oil

**8 asparagus spears,
cut into 1–2in
(2.5–5cm) pieces**

2 eggs

**1 tbsp milk or plant-based
alternative**

1 tsp dried dill

**7.4oz (210g) can salmon
(about 7oz/200g drained
weight), or 1 salmon
fillet, poached**

**2 handfuls of watercress,
to serve**

**supports weight management • helps reduce
inflammation • supports early fetal development**

A classic combo, eggs and salmon deliver on protein to satisfy the appetite. Anti-inflammatory omega-3 in salmon may be especially helpful for egg quality in women in their mid- to late-thirties onwards, referred to as an advanced maternal age. Salmon also supplies choline and iodine, supporting fetal development.

Heat the oil in a deep skillet over medium heat. Once hot, add the asparagus spears and cook for 2–3 minutes, until the asparagus is starting to brown.

Place the eggs and milk in a small bowl and whisk with a fork, then sprinkle in the dill and stir to combine. Arrange the asparagus pieces so they are spread out evenly in the pan, then pour the egg mixture into the pan and swirl to coat the base.

Gently flake the salmon over the top. Cover with a lid and cook for 7–10 minutes, until the egg has set. Cut the frittata in half and serve with a side of watercress.

Salmon *with* beet *and* cottage cheese *on* toast

Makes 2
Prep 5 mins

1 cooked beet, diced
2 tbsp cottage cheese
pinch of freshly ground
black pepper
squeeze of lemon juice, plus
lemon wedges to serve
2 slices whole wheat bread
or multigrain crispbreads
1 salmon fillet (about 7oz/
200g), poached and flaked
handful of microgreens
4 walnuts, crushed

has anti-inflammatory properties • may support implantation • supports uterine health

This simple snack is nutritionally dense. Salmon and walnuts supply anti-inflammatory omega-3s while beets add fiber and nitrates, supporting blood flow to the uterus and, in turn, improving the chances of implantation.

Place the beet, cottage cheese, pepper, and lemon juice in a small bowl and mix together.

If having on toast, lightly toast the bread. Spoon the beet mixture on top of the toast or crispbread and top with the poached salmon. Add the pea shoots and walnuts and serve with lemon wedges.

114

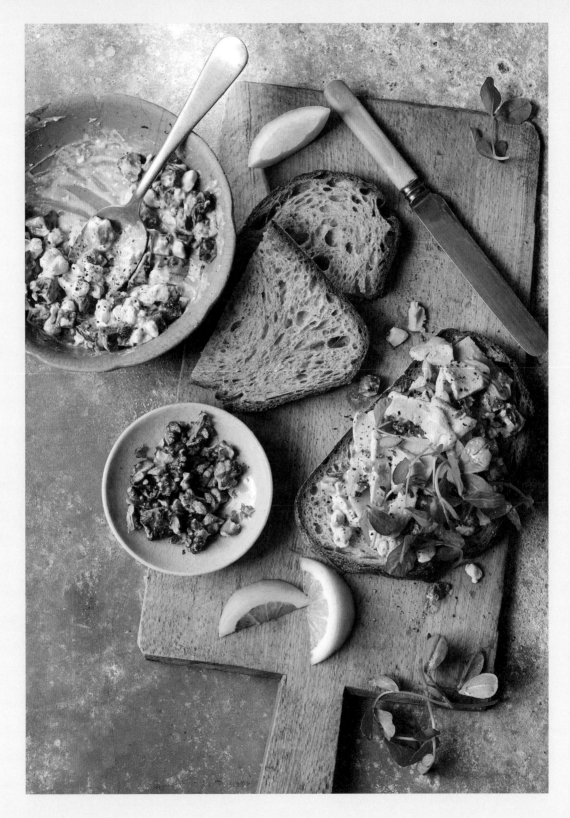

Salmon with beet and cottage cheese on toast

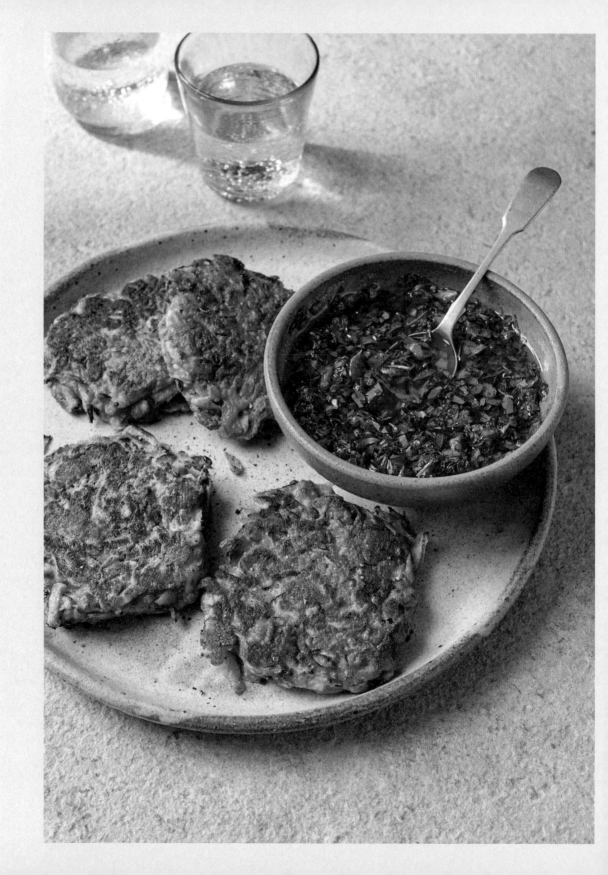

Zucchini fritters
and salsa verde

Serves 2
Prep 5 mins
Cook 20 mins, plus cooling

2 eggs, whisked
¹/₂ cup (65g) whole wheat
   self-rising flour
1 zucchini, grated (squeezed
   and excess liquid drained
   through a sieve)
1 carrot, grated (squeezed
   and excess liquid drained
   through a sieve)
1oz (30g) feta, crumbled
1 tsp smoked paprika
handful of mint leaves, chopped
1 tbsp olive oil

For the salsa verde
1 garlic clove, diced
handful of flat-leaf parsley
   leaves, chopped
handful of basil leaves, chopped
handful of mint leaves, chopped
1 tsp red wine vinegar
juice of ¹/₄ lemon
1–2 tbsp extra-virgin olive oil
1 tsp capers
¹/₂ green chile, diced

promotes hormonal balance • may help reduce conception time • aids egg and sperm health • may support implantation

Refreshing zucchinis supply antioxidant vitamin C, good levels of which are thought to support progesterone and favorable conception times. Olive oil adds vitamin E to promote egg and sperm health and support implantation.

Place the egg and flour in a bowl and mix together well. Add the zucchini, carrot, feta, paprika, and mint and combine.

Heat the oil in a skillet over medium heat. Add a large spoonful—about a quarter—of the zucchini mixture to the frying pan and fry for 2–3 minutes on each side, until golden and heated through. Remove from the pan and keep the fritter warm while you cook the remaining 3 fritters.

In the meantime, mix together all the ingredients for the salsa verde. Serve the hot fritters alongside the salsa verde.

Lima bean *and* vegetable soup

Serves 2
Prep 5 mins
Cook 35 mins

1 tbsp vegetable oil
1 potato, peeled and diced
1 carrot, sliced
½ onion, diced
2 celery stalks, diced
1 garlic clove, finely
   chopped
1 tsp dried oregano
14oz (400g) can of lima
   beans, drained and rinsed
16fl oz (500ml) reduced-salt
   vegetable stock
2 handfuls of kale or
   spinach, roughly chopped
1 tsp lemon juice
handful of flat-leaf parsley,
   chopped
2 tsp Parmesan cheese,
   grated
whole wheat toast, with
   olive-based spread if
   desired, to serve

Flex it—*Omit Parmesan cheese for a vegan soup. Replace with a nondairy alternative if desired.*

supplies fiber • promotes hormonal balance • supports ovulatory health

This warming soup has fiber and low GI carbs to help regulate blood sugar levels, insulin, and other hormones. Lima beans also supply iron and folate, supporting ovulation.

Heat the oil in a lidded saucepan over medium heat. Once hot, add the potato, carrot, onion, celery, garlic, and oregano. Cook for 5 minutes, stirring frequently.

Add the lima beans to the pan. Cook, stirring, for another 2 minutes, then add the stock and bring to a boil. Lower the heat, partially cover the pan, and simmer for 20–30 minutes.

Add the kale or spinach leaves during the final 5 minutes of the cooking time. Stir in the lemon juice and parsley, ladle the soup into 2 bowls, and sprinkle with the Parmesan cheese. Serve with whole wheat toast, buttered, if desired, with oil-based spread.

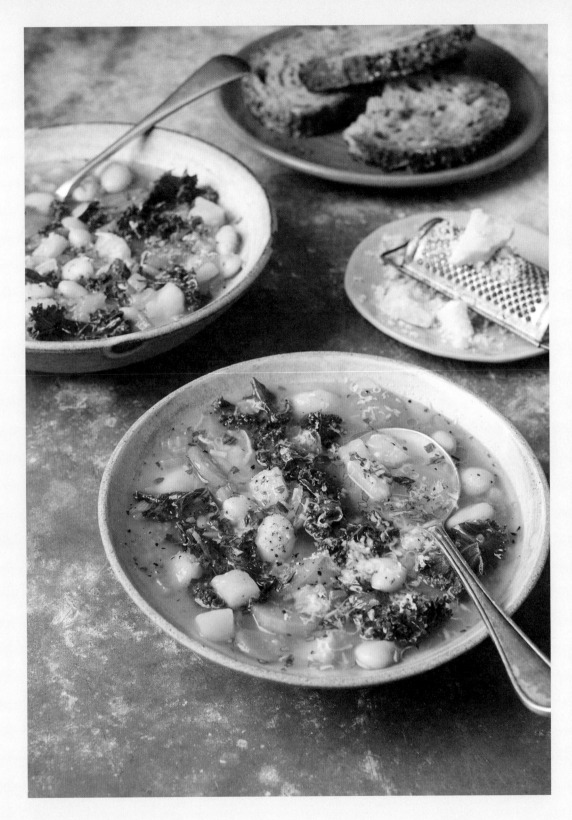

Lima bean and vegetable soup

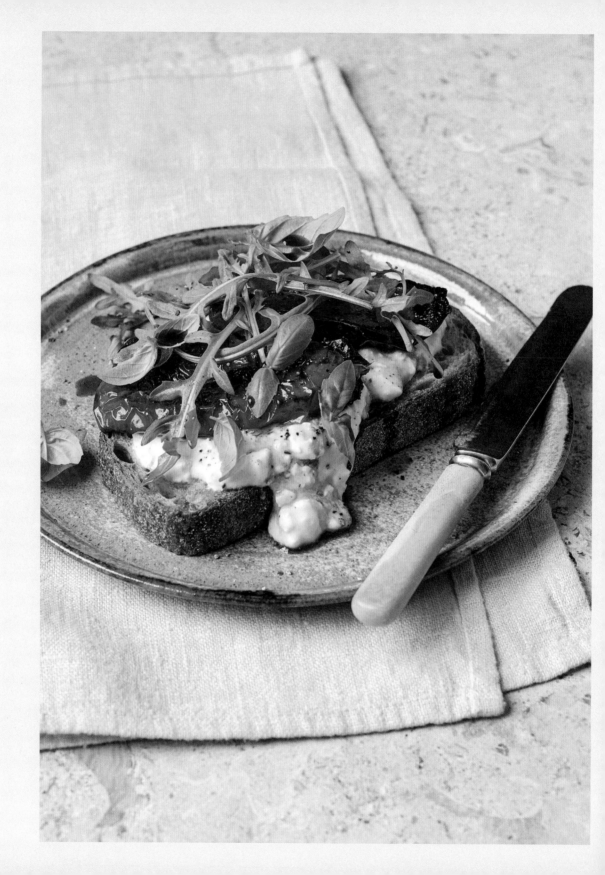

Red pepper *and* cottage cheese toast

provides antioxidants • promotes hormonal balance

With deliciously sweet and tender grilled peppers and creamy cottage cheese, this simple bite is a must-have! Peppers are high in antioxidant vitamin C, thought to support progesterone levels. Cottage cheese adds essential protein as well as fertility-promoting selenium and vitamin B12.

Serves 1
Prep 5 mins
Cook 10 mins

1/2 **red pepper, seeded and halved**
1 tsp olive oil
1–2 slices of whole wheat bread
2 tbsp cottage cheese
handful of arugula
pinch of salt and freshly ground black pepper
handful of basil leaves, to garnish
1/2 **tsp balsamic vinegar**

Preheat the grill to medium-hot. Brush the peppers with the olive oil and grill for 10 minutes, until the skin begins to blister.

Lightly toast the bread. Top the toast with the cottage cheese, red pepper, and arugula, and season. Garnish with the basil leaves, drizzle over the balsamic vinegar, and enjoy right away.

Edamame noodle salad

Serves 2
Prep 5 mins
Cook 10 mins

²/₃ cup (100g) shelled edamame beans
2 nests of whole wheat noodles
handful of bean sprouts
4 radishes, sliced
¼ cucumber, cut into ribbons
2 scallions, sliced
juice of 1 lime
1 tsp low-sodium soy sauce
1 tbsp extra-virgin olive oil
1 tbsp cashews, crushed
handful of Thai basil leaves

hydrates • supports ovulatory health • may support implantation • may support fertility treatments

Refreshing and flavorsome, this has plant-based protein, from cashews and edamame beans, to aid ovulation; and whole grains to support implantation.

Place a saucepan of water over a medium-high heat and bring to a boil. Add the edamame beans and cook for about 5 minutes, according to the package instructions. Drain and set aside to cool.

Place another saucepan of water over a medium-high heat. Bring to a boil, add the noodle nests, and cook until softened. Drain and rinse under cold water.

Place the noodles in a large bowl. Add the edamame beans and remaining ingredients and mix thoroughly to combine. Spoon into 2 bowls and enjoy cold.

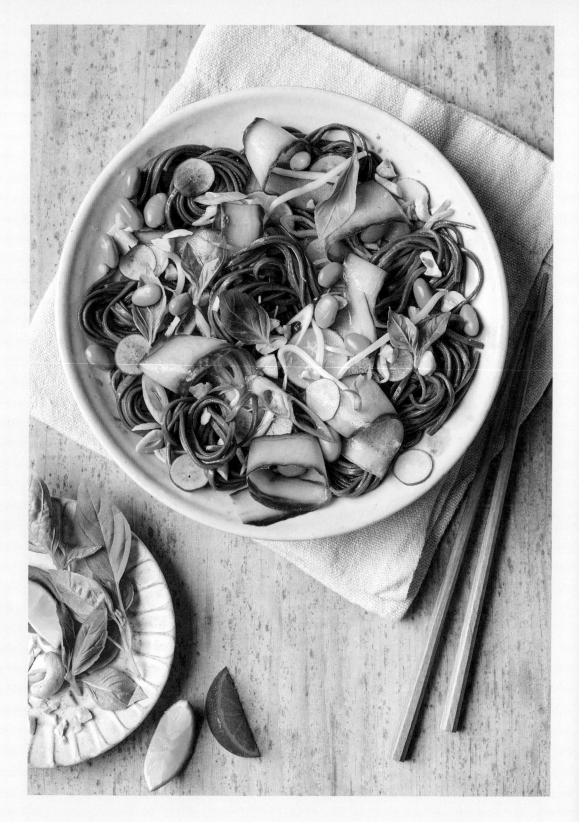

Edamame noodle salad

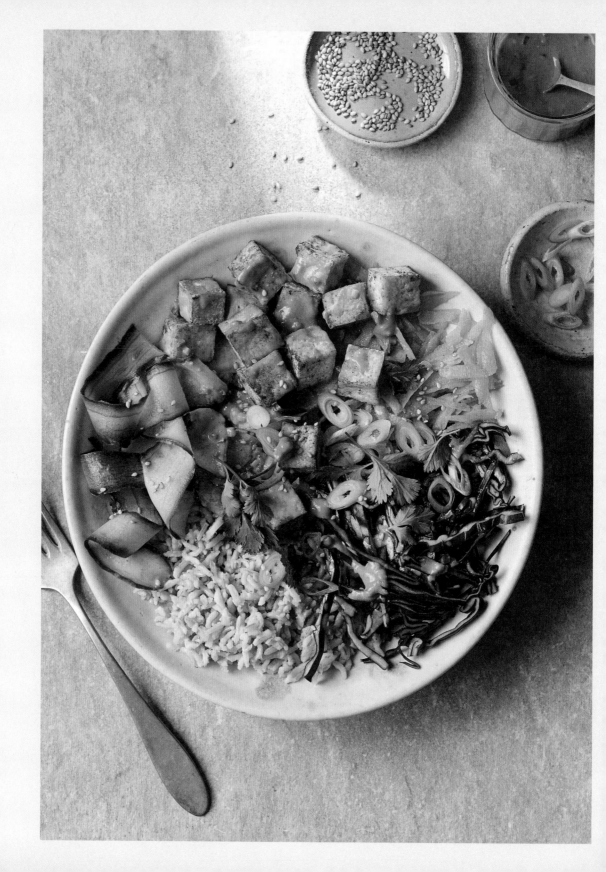

Tofu satay *with* crunchy rainbow salad

Serves 2
Prep 5 mins
Cook 25 mins

¾ cup (150g) brown rice
1 tsp vegetable oil
1 block extra-firm tofu, drained, rinsed, and diced into 1in (2.5cm) pieces
1 tsp ground cinnamon
1 carrot, grated
¼ red cabbage, shredded
½ cucumber, cut into ribbons
1 scallion, sliced
juice of 1 lime
1 tsp sesame oil
1 tsp sesame seeds
handful of cilantro leaves, chopped, to garnish

For the satay sauce
1 tbsp low-sodium soy sauce
1 tbsp unsalted smooth peanut butter
1 tsp rice wine vinegar
1 tsp lime juice
1 tsp sesame oil
½ tsp curry powder
½ red chile, seeded and diced
1in (2.5cm) piece of ginger, diced
1 garlic clove, diced

supports ovulatory health • provides antioxidants • promotes hormonal balance

A high-quality plant protein, tofu supports healthy ovulation, while whole grain brown rice has a low GI ranking, helping to steady blood sugars, insulin, and other hormones. The colorful salad adds a host of fertility-promoting antioxidants.

Bring a lidded saucepan of water to a boil. Add the rice, reduce the heat to a simmer, and cook, covered, for 15–20 minutes, or according to the package instructions. Place all the ingredients for the satay sauce in a bowl and mix to combine.

In the meantime, heat the vegetable oil in a skillet over medium-high heat. Once hot, add the tofu and cinnamon. Fry the tofu for 3 minutes each side, until slightly browned.

Reduce the heat of the tofu pan to low and add the satay sauce. Cook for 5 minutes, stirring continuously. Add a splash of water if the mixture becomes too thick.

Divide the tofu and the rice between 2 bowls. Add the carrot, red cabbage, cucumber, and scallion, drizzle over the lime juice and sesame oil, and top with the sesame seeds. Drizzle over any leftover satay sauce and garnish with cilantro.

Mackerel *and* beet potato salad

Serves 2
Prep 5 mins
Cook 10–15 mins

6–8 new potatoes, thinly sliced
2 tbsp crème fraîche
1 tbsp dried dill
½ tsp Dijon mustard
juice of ½ lemon
1 tsp capers
¼ cucumber, diced
2 radishes, diced
1 celery stalk, diced
1 scallion, diced
1 beet, thinly sliced
handful of flat-leaf parsley
   leaves, chopped
2 cooked mackerel fillets,
   skin removed
2 handfuls of watercress,
   to serve

provides antioxidants • supplies fiber • has anti-inflammatory properties • aids egg and sperm health

A medley of flavors and nutrients, this scrumptious salad has fiber-rich veggies for gut health. Radishes, celery, scallions, and potatoes also supply vitamin C, to support progesterone. Mackerel adds anti-inflammatory omega-3, for egg and sperm health.

Place the potatoes in a saucepan of boiling water and cook for 10–15 minutes, until soft. Drain and rinse under cold water.

Place the crème fraîche, dill, mustard, and lemon juice in a bowl and mix together. Place the potatoes in a serving bowl, then add the capers, cucumber, radishes, celery, scallion, beet, and parsley. Scoop in the crème fraîche mixture and stir to combine.

Flake the mackerel into the serving bowl and serve the potato salad with a side of watercress.

Fig, feta, *and* barley salad

Serves 2
Prep 5 mins
Cook 30 mins

¹/₃ cup (70g) pearl barley
handful of arugula
handful of spinach
handful of mint leaves,
 chopped
1 tbsp pomegranate seeds
4 Brazil nuts, roughly
 chopped
2 figs, quartered
1oz (30g) feta, diced

For the dressing
1 scallion, finely chopped
1 tsp lemon juice
1 tbsp extra-virgin
 olive oil
1 tsp balsamic vinegar
¹/₂ tsp Dijon mustard

supplies fiber and folate • aids egg and sperm health • supports gut health

Honey-sweet figs are full of fiber, supporting gut health, while Brazil nuts are an excellent source of the antioxidant selenium, supporting egg and sperm quality. Feta is a source of essential folate.

Place the pearl barley in a lidded saucepan, cover with water, and bring to a boil. Reduce the heat to a simmer, cover, and cook for 25–30 minutes, according to the package instructions. Drain if needed and set aside.

Place the arugula, spinach, mint leaves, pomegranate seeds, Brazil nuts, figs, and feta in a large bowl.

To make the dressing, stir all the ingredients together. Combine the pearl barley with the salad, pour over the dressing, and toss everything together to combine. Enjoy warm.

(photographed overleaf)

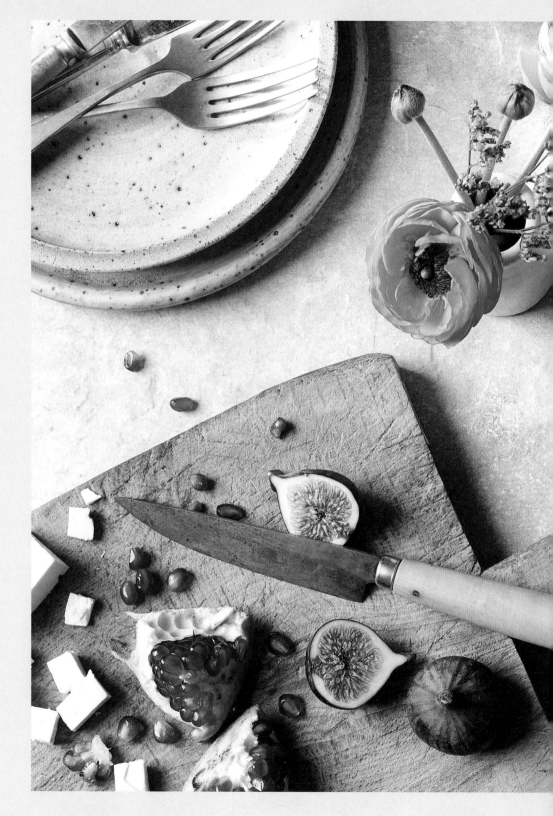

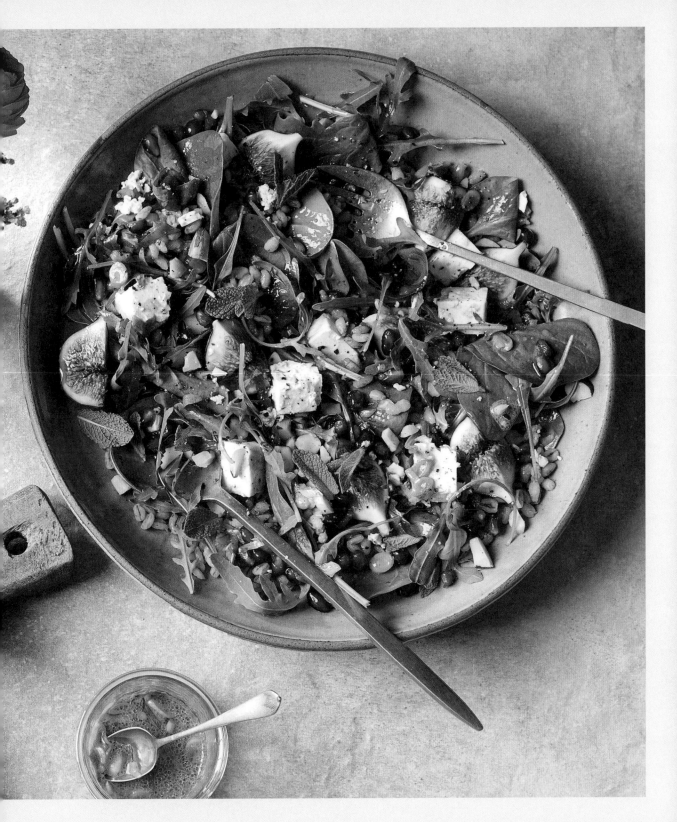

Fig, feta, and barley salad

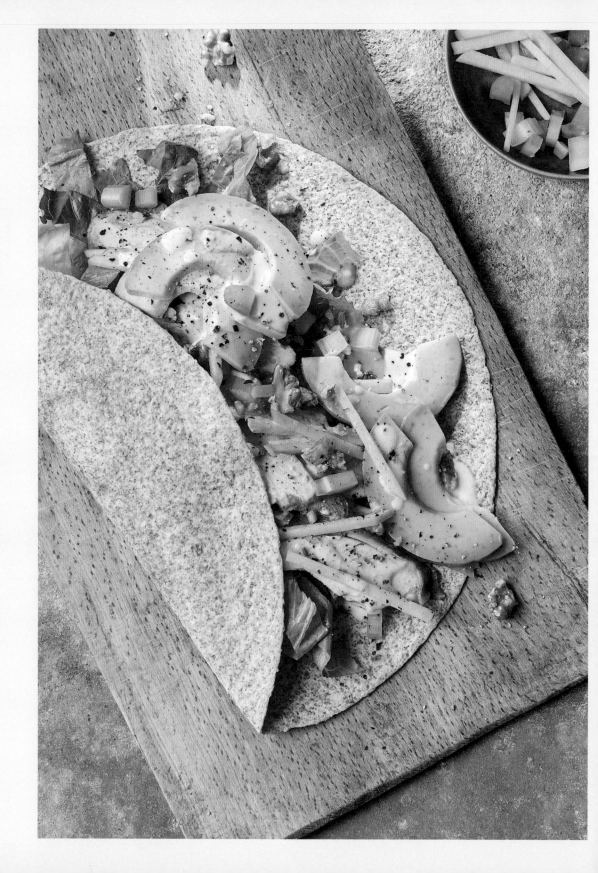

Chicken, avocado, *and* walnut wrap

Serves 1

Prep 5 mins

1 tbsp Greek yogurt
juice of ¼ lemon
½ tsp Dijon mustard
4½oz (125g) **chicken,**
    cooked and cut into strips
3 **walnuts, crumbled**
1 **celery stalk, diced**
½ **apple, cored and cut**
    into matchsticks
½ **avocado, pitted and**
    sliced
1 **scallion, diced**
pinch of freshly ground
    black pepper
2 **romaine lettuce leaves,**
    sliced
1 **whole wheat tortilla wrap**

Flex it—*For a veggie wrap,
swap in 4½oz (125g) cooked tofu
in place of the chicken.*

**has anti-inflammatory properties • aids egg
and sperm health • supplies fiber**

This delicious wrap is an all-in-one bundle of
fertility-promoting nutrients. Chicken has vital
protein, selenium, and vitamin B6; walnuts supply
omega-3s; and apples add fiber, linked to higher
conception rates.

Place the yogurt, lemon juice, and mustard in a small
bowl and stir to combine. Add the chicken, walnuts,
celery, apple, avocado, and scallion, and season with
black pepper.

Place the lettuce on the wrap, spoon the filling in a line
down the middle of the wrap, and roll the wrap around
the filling. Enjoy!

Eggplant *with* pistachio *and* pomegranate freekeh

Serves 2
Prep 10 mins
Cook 40 mins

1 eggplant, cut in half
    lengthwise
1 tbsp olive oil
1 tbsp harissa paste
¹/₂ cup (80g) freekeh (or
    buckwheat if preferred),
    rinsed under cold water
2 handfuls of salad leaves
2 small beet, sliced
¹/₄ cucumber, sliced
handful of flat-leaf parsley,
    chopped
1 tbsp pomegranate seeds
1 tbsp pistachios, chopped

For the tahini sauce
1 tbsp tahini
1 tsp lemon juice
1 tbsp yogurt
1 tsp extra-virgin olive oil
1 tsp sumac or lemon
    pepper

**supports healthy ovulation • aids egg
and sperm health**

The ever-popular eggplant is full of fiber,
supporting gut health and ovulation. Freekeh and
pistachios supply plant-based proteins, to support
ovulation, while olive oil has vitamin E, promoting
both egg and sperm quality.

Preheat the oven to 400°F (180°C). Score the flesh of
the eggplant halves with a sharp knife then coat them
in the olive oil and harissa paste. Place the eggplants
on a baking sheet and roast for 40 minutes.

In the meantime, add the freekeh or buckwheat to a
saucepan with 7fl oz (200ml) of boiling water. Reduce
the heat to a simmer and cook for 20–30 minutes (or
about 10 minutes if using buckwheat), or according
to the package instructions.

Place the salad leaves, beet, cucumber, parsley,
pomegranate seeds, pistachios, and the freekeh
or buckwheat in a large bowl and toss to combine.

To make the tahini sauce, stir together all the
ingredients. Serve the roasted eggplant on top of
the freekeh salad and spoon over the tahini sauce.

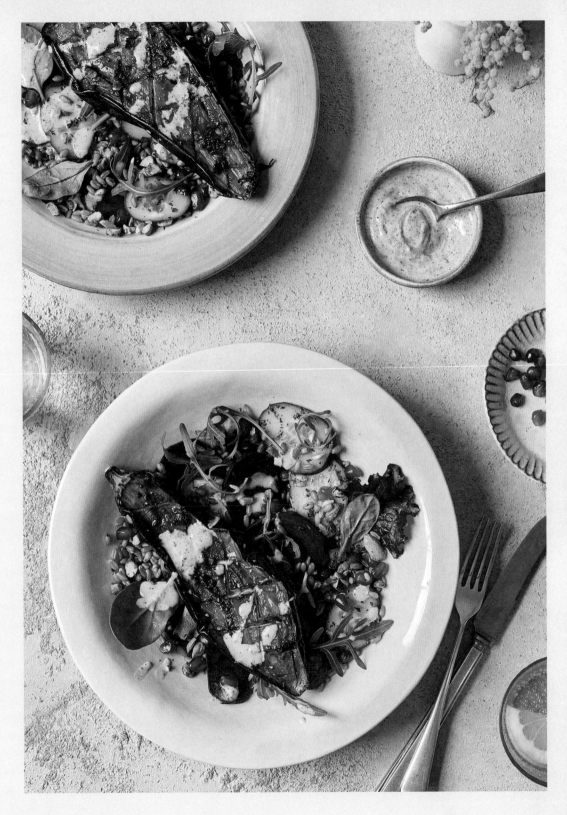

Eggplant with pistachio and pomegranate freekeh

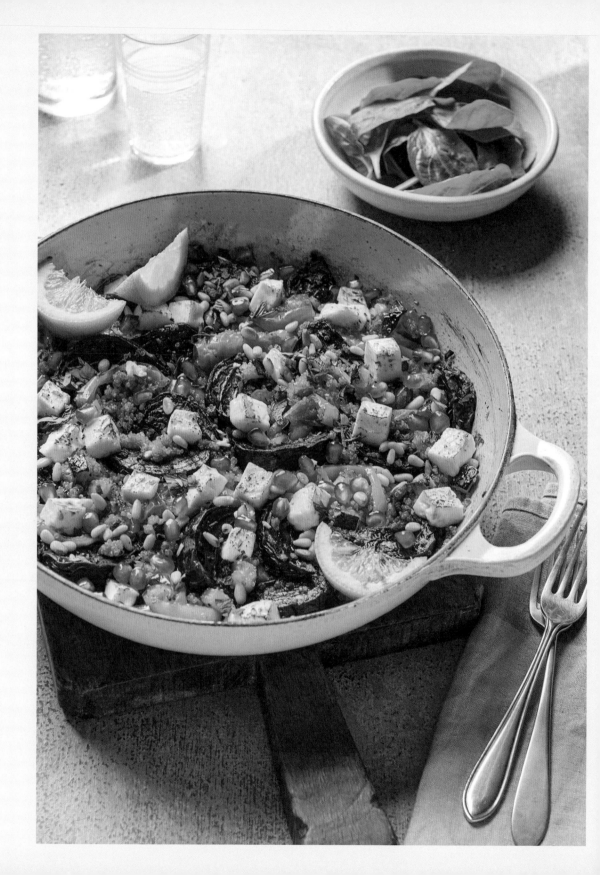

Jeweled quinoa

Serves 2
Prep 5 mins
Cook 30–35 mins

1 garlic clove, thinly sliced
2 beets, cut into wedges
1 orange pepper, seeded
  and cut into strips
¼ zucchini, diced
10 cherry tomatoes, halved
1 tbsp olive oil
⅓ cup (60g) dried quinoa,
  rinsed under cold water
  several times
14fl oz (400ml) low-sodium
  vegetable stock
2oz (60g) feta, cut into
  ½in (1cm) cubes
1 tbsp pine nuts
handful of cilantro leaves,
  chopped
handful of mint leaves,
  chopped
1 tbsp pomegranate seeds
2 large handfuls of spinach,
  to serve
lemon wedges, to serve

may support progesterone levels • may support implantation

Peppers and pomegranates are high in progesterone-supporting vitamin C. Beets contain nitrates, which convert to nitric oxide in the body; this compound dilates blood vessels, facilitating healthy blood flow to the uterus.

Preheat the oven to 425°F (200°C). Place the garlic, beets, orange pepper, zucchini, and tomatoes in an ovenproof dish and drizzle over the olive oil. Put the dish in the oven and roast for 25–30 minutes.

In the meantime, place the quinoa in a lidded saucepan with the stock. Bring to a boil, then reduce the heat to a simmer, cover, and cook for 10–15 minutes, or according to the package instructions, until the quinoa has softened and the liquid has been absorbed.

Remove the dish from the oven and stir in the quinoa. Preheat the grill to medium-high. Arrange the feta and pine nuts on top of the quinoa mixture, then place under the grill for 5 minutes. Remove and top with the cilantro, mint, and pomegranate seeds. Serve with spinach and lemon wedges. If batch cooking, keep covered in the fridge for up to 3 days. Or place the quinoa and vegetable mixture (without the cheese) in an airtight container and freeze for up to 3 months.

Chickpea shakshuka

Serves 2
Prep 5–10 mins
Cook 25 mins

1 tbsp olive oil
$^1/_2$ red onion, diced
1 red pepper, seeded and
   diced
1 garlic clove, finely chopped
1 tsp smoked paprika
1 tsp ground cumin
$^1/_2$ tsp ground coriander
$^1/_2$ tsp ground cinnamon
$^1/_4$ tsp cayenne pepper
14fl oz (400ml) tomato puree,
   ideally from a glass jar
6 cherry tomatoes, halved
13.4oz (380g) carton of
   chickpeas, drained and
   rinsed
pinch of salt
juice of $^1/_4$ lemon
2 eggs
handful of cilantro leaves,
   chopped, to garnish
2 mini whole wheat pita
   breads, toasted, to serve
   (optional)

aids sperm health • supports healthy ovulation • provides key antioxidants • supplies iron

This flavorsome dish is high in antioxidants such as vitamin C. Tomatoes also supply lycopene, thought to promote healthy sperm, and chickpeas are a good source of plant-based protein and iron, key ovulation-supporting nutrients.

Heat the oil in a lidded saucepan or deep skillet over medium heat. Once hot, add the onion and red pepper and fry for 5 minutes. Add the garlic, paprika, cumin, coriander, cinnamon, and cayenne pepper and stir to coat the vegetables in the spices.

Pour in the tomato puree and add the cherry tomatoes, chickpeas, a pinch of salt, and the lemon juice. Bring to a boil, then reduce the heat and simmer for 10 minutes. Make 2 wells in the mixture and gently crack an egg into each hole. Cover and cook for 5–8 minutes, until the eggs are cooked through. Garnish with the cilantro leaves and serve with pita bread, if desired.

If batch cooking, omit the eggs and fry them when ready to serve. Keep the chickpea mixture in an airtight container in the fridge for up to 3 days or freeze for up to 3 months.

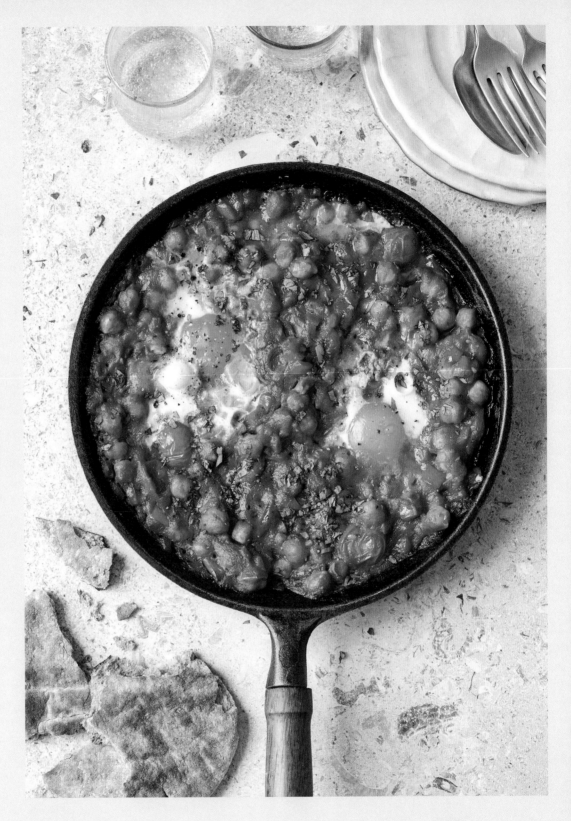

Chickpea shakshuka

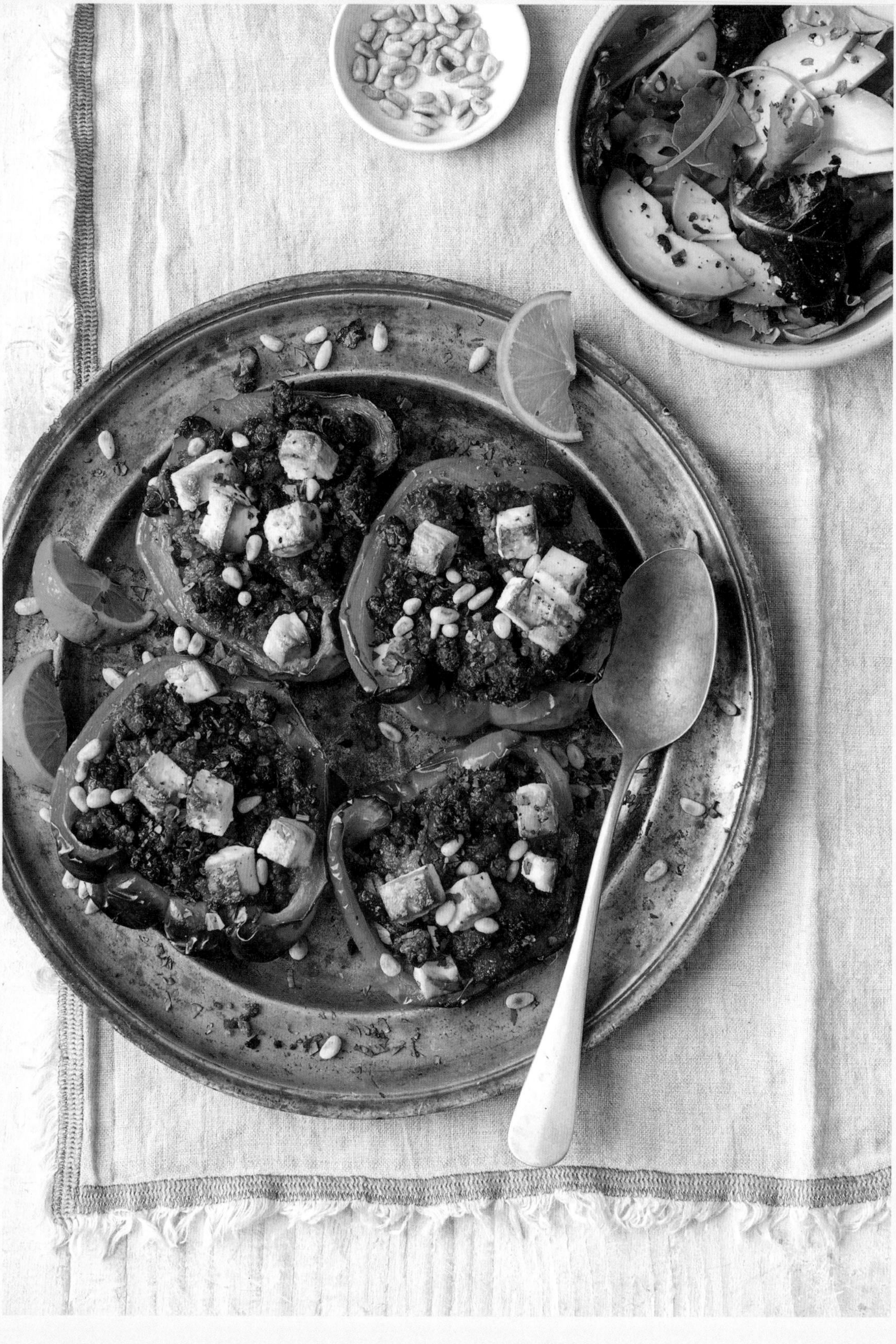

Quinoa-stuffed peppers

Serves 2
Prep 5 mins
Cook 35–40 mins

¹/₃ cup (60g) dried quinoa, rinsed
    under cold water several times
6fl oz (180ml) low-sodium
    vegetable stock
1 tbsp olive oil
¹/₂ onion, diced
1 garlic clove, finely chopped
13.4oz (380g) carton of black
    beans, drained and rinsed
3¹/₂fl oz (100ml) tomato puree,
    ideally from a glass jar
1 large tomato, diced
¹/₄ tsp cayenne pepper
1 tsp smoked paprika
¹/₂ tsp ground cumin
2 red peppers, seeded and
    cut in half lengthwise
1oz (30g) feta, cut into ¹/₂in
    (1cm) cubes
handful of cilantro leaves,
    chopped, to garnish
1 tbsp pine nuts, to garnish
lime wedges, to serve

For the salad
handful of salad leaves
1 avocado, pitted and sliced
¹/₂ tsp chili flakes, to serve

**provides antioxidants • promotes hormonal
balance • supports healthy ovulation**

This antioxidant-rich dish is filled with flavor.
Quinoa and black beans provide plant-based protein,
promoting healthy ovulation. They also supply
fiber, helping to steady blood sugars, insulin,
and other hormones.

Preheat the oven to 425°F (200°C). Put the quinoa
in a lidded saucepan with the stock. Bring to a boil,
reduce to a simmer, cover, and cook for 10–15 minutes,
or according to the package instructions, until the
quinoa has softened and the liquid is absorbed. In
the meantime, heat the oil in a large saucepan over
medium heat. Add the onion, cook for 5 minutes, then
add the garlic and cook for 1 minute. Add the black
beans, tomato puree, tomato, cayenne, paprika, and
cumin, and simmer for 5 minutes. Stir in the cooked
quinoa.

Place the red peppers on a baking sheet, cut-side up,
and fill evenly with the quinoa mixture. Top with the
feta and bake for 25 minutes. Garnish with the cilantro
and pine nuts. Serve with lime wedges and a side of
salad leaves topped with avocado and chili flakes.

Flex it—*Swap the black beans for 9oz (250g) lean ground beef.
Add to the pan after the onions and garlic and cook for 5 minutes
until brown, then continue with the recipe.*

Buckwheat *and* beet salad

Serves 2
Prep 5 mins
Cook 5–10 mins, plus cooling

1 cup (150g) buckwheat, rinsed
8 asparagus spears, halved
handful of broccolini, cut into
   small florets
2 cooked beets, thinly sliced
   or grated
1 avocado, diced
$\frac{1}{2}$ cup (80g) edamame beans
1 tbsp sunflower seeds
4 Brazil nuts or small handful
   of peanuts, roughly chopped
2 handfuls of spinach
pinch of salt and freshly
   ground black pepper
handful of mint leaves,
   chopped

For the dressing
2 tbsp extra-virgin olive oil
1 tsp balsamic vinegar
juice of $\frac{1}{2}$ lemon

aids egg health • has anti-inflammatory properties • supports early fetal development

This refreshing salad is rich in folate from the asparagus, broccolini, beets, and edamame beans. Folate aids egg health and is key in early pregnancy. Brazil nuts add healthy anti-inflammatory fats and selenium, helpful for women's reproductive health.

Add the buckwheat to a saucepan and cover with water. Bring to a boil, then reduce the heat to a simmer and cook for 5–10 minutes, or according to the package instructions, until tender. Drain any excess water and let the buckwheat cool slightly.

Steam the asparagus and broccolini. Place the beets, avocado, edamame beans, sunflower seeds, Brazil nuts or peanuts, spinach, salt and pepper, and the mint leaves in a large bowl. Stir to combine.

To make the dressing, place the ingredients in a small bowl and whisk together. Add the buckwheat, asparagus, and broccolini to the salad bowl, pour over the dressing, and toss to combine. Enjoy right away.

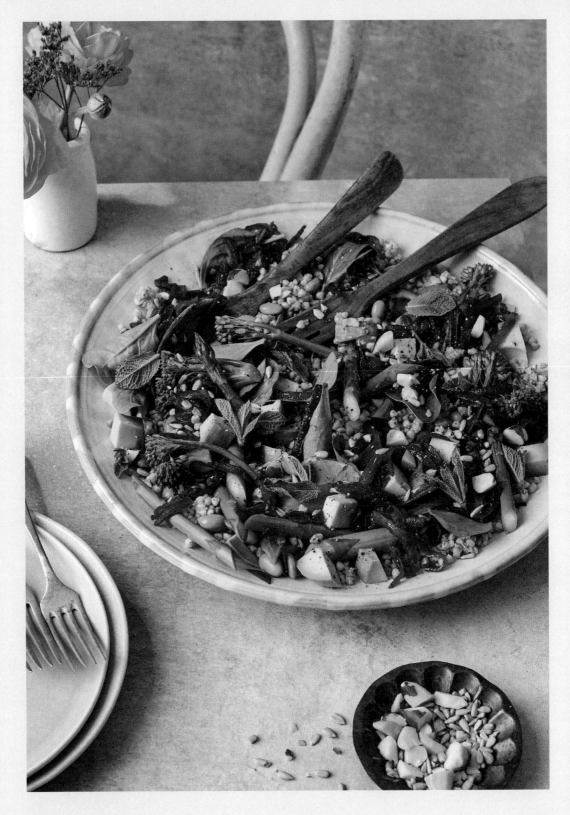

Buckwheat and beet salad

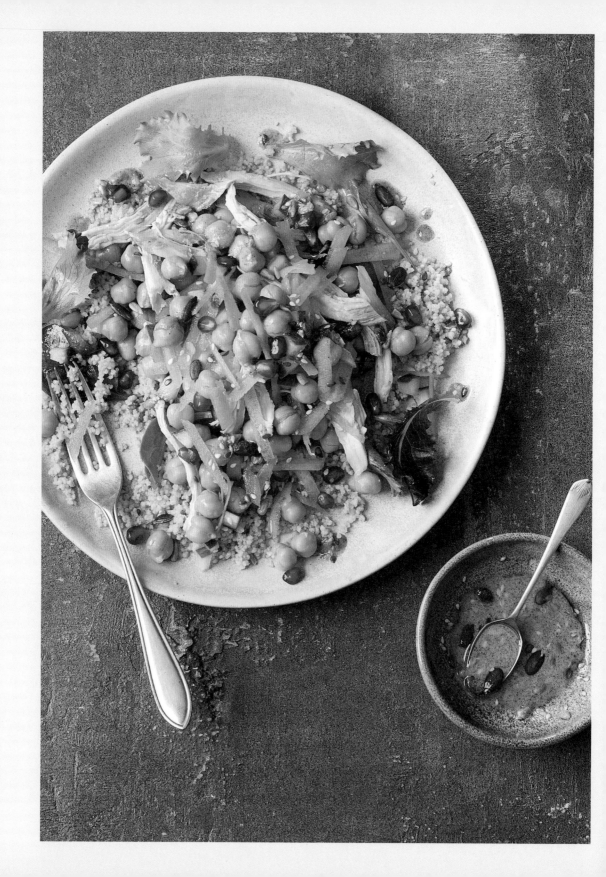

Chicken, chickpea, *and* couscous salad

Serves 2
Prep 5 mins
Cook 5–10 mins

$^1/_3$ cup (60g) whole wheat
    couscous
2 handfuls of salad leaves
    or spinach
10oz (300g) chicken breast,
    cooked and shredded
13.4oz (380g) carton of
    chickpeas, drained and
    rinsed
5 cucumber slices, diced
1 carrot, grated
handful of mint leaves,
    chopped (optional)
1 tbsp pomegranate seeds

For the dressing
1 tbsp extra-virgin olive oil
1 tbsp mixed seeds
$^1/_4$ tsp ground cinnamon
$^1/_2$ tsp ground cumin
1 tsp lemon juice
$^1/_2$ tsp **Dijon mustard**

**supplies iron and folate • aids egg and sperm
health • supports healthy ovulation**

This appetizing chicken and chickpea combo
delivers essential protein and iron, crucial for
the healthy development of eggs and sperm and
supporting healthy ovulation. Juicy pomegranates
add folate and the antioxidant vitamin C.

Place the couscous in a bowl and pour over freshly
boiled water to just cover it. Cover the couscous with
a plate or lid and leave for 5–10 minutes to soften,
then fluff it up with a fork.

In the meantime, place all of the ingredients for the
dressing in a small bowl and mix together. Place the
salad leaves or spinach, chicken, chickpeas, cucumber,
carrot, mint (if desired), and pomegranate seeds in a
large bowl and toss to combine. Spoon the couscous
onto 2 plates, top with the chicken and chickpea salad,
pour over the dressing, and serve immediately.

Tomato, broccolini, *and* mozzarella pasta

Serves 2
Prep 5–10 mins
Cook 15 mins

5¹/₂oz (150g) whole wheat
   pasta of choice
1 tbsp olive oil
¹/₂ red onion, diced
handful of broccolini, florets
   and stems, cut into small
   pieces
¹/₂ green pepper, seeded and
   diced
1 garlic clove, finely chopped
2oz (60g) mozzarella, torn
   into small pieces
10 sun-dried tomatoes,
   chopped
10 black olives, pitted
   and halved
1 tbsp pesto
1 tbsp pine nuts
2 handfuls of basil leaves
2 handfuls of arugula, to
   serve

**provides antioxidants • supplies folate
• supports early fetal development • has
anti-inflammatory properties**

This taste of the Mediterranean is full of antioxidants, promoting healthy egg and sperm. Broccolini adds folate, supporting fertility and early pregnancy, while the olives provide anti-inflammatory unsaturated fats and antioxidant vitamin E.

Place the pasta in a saucepan of boiling water and cook for 10 minutes, or according to the package instructions. Set aside a small cupful of the pasta water before draining.

In the meantime, heat the oil in a skillet over medium heat. Once hot, add the onion, broccolini, green pepper, and garlic and cook for 5–10 minutes, stirring regularly. Reduce the heat to low, then add the mozzarella, sun-dried tomatoes, olives, pesto, the cooked pasta, and the reserved pasta cooking water. Stir to combine for 1–2 minutes, until all the ingredients are heated through.

Spoon the pasta into 2 bowls, top with the pine nuts and basil, and serve with a side of arugula.

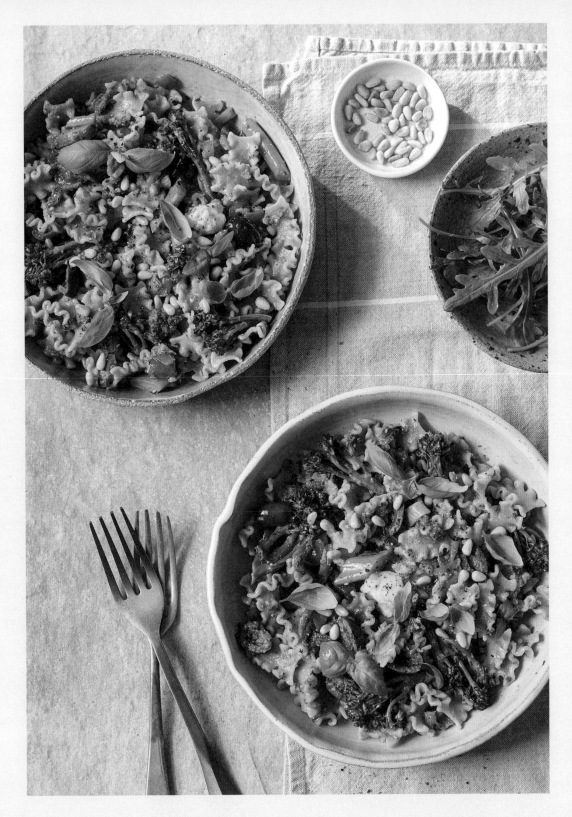

Tomato, broccolini, and mozzarella pasta

145

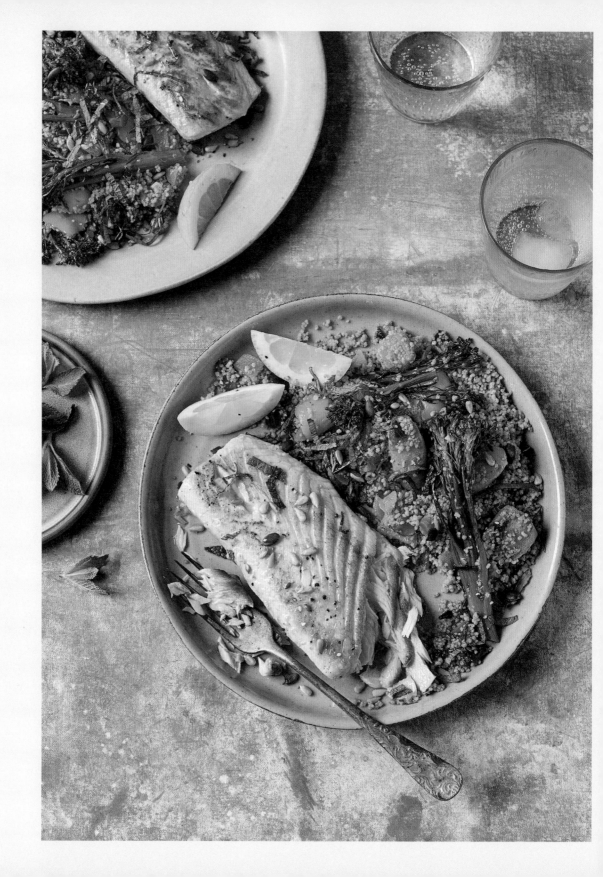

Salmon *with* harissa vegetable couscous

Serves 2
Prep 5 mins
Cook 30 mins

1 carrot, sliced diagonally
1 orange pepper, seeded
    and diced
handful of broccolini
$\frac{1}{2}$ red onion, diced
1 garlic clove, sliced
1 tsp harissa paste
2 tbsp olive oil, divided
1 tsp ground cumin
2 salmon fillets, about 5oz
    (140g) each
$\frac{1}{2}$ cup (70g) whole wheat
    couscous
juice and zest of $\frac{1}{2}$ orange
$\frac{1}{2}$ tsp ground cinnamon
1 tbsp dried apricots, diced
1 tbsp mixed seeds
handful of mint leaves, chopped
lemon wedges, to serve

provides antioxidants • aids egg health

This colorful dish is rich in antioxidants, thought to be especially helpful for those undergoing fertility treatment. Salmon is high in omega-3s, which promote egg health, especially in women in their mid- to late-thirties onwards, seen as an advanced maternal age.

Preheat the oven to 400°F (180°C). Parboil the carrot for 5 minutes, until softened slightly. Place the carrot, orange pepper, broccolini, red onion, garlic, harissa, 1 tablespoon of the oil, and the cumin on a baking sheet, toss to mix thoroughly, and roast for 20–30 minutes.

In the final 10 minutes of the vegetable cooking time, heat the remaining oil in a large, lidded skillet over medium-high heat. Once hot, add the salmon fillets, skin-side down. Cover and cook for about 10 minutes, turning halfway through, until the salmon is cooked through, opaque, and flakes easily when cut with a knife.

In the last 5 minutes of the vegetable cooking, put the couscous, orange juice and zest, cinnamon, and apricots in a bowl and pour over 2½fl oz (70ml) of just-boiled water. Cover with a plate for 5 minutes, then use a fork to separate and fluff the grains. Add the couscous to the vegetables, with the seeds and mint leaves, and stir to combine. Serve the harissa vegetable couscous alongside the salmon, with lemon wedges on the side.

Prawn poke bowl

Serves 2
Prep 10 mins
Marinate 15–60 mins
Cook 15–20 mins

juice of 1 lime
½ chile, seeded and finely
  diced
2 tbsp extra-virgin olive oil
7oz (200g) cooked and
  peeled prawns
¾ cup (150g) brown rice
2 carrots, grated
1 cooked beet, diced
½ cucumber, grated
2 scallions, sliced
2 radishes, thinly sliced
handful of cilantro leaves
1 tbsp black sesame seeds
½ tsp chili flakes
pinch of salt

Flex it—*For a vegan dish,
swap the prawns for 1 block
of cooked tofu or 3½oz (100g)
cooked edamame beans, added
to the bowl with the other salad
items. Pour the marinade over
before serving.*

aids egg and sperm health • supplies fiber • provides antioxidants

Tasty and quick to prep, this dish delivers vitamin B12 and zinc from the succulent prawns, to support sperm volume, concentration, and motility. Brightly colored vegetables and whole grain brown rice add fiber and an array of fertility-promoting antioxidants.

Place the lime juice, chile, and olive oil in a small bowl and combine. Add the prawns and let marinate for 15–60 minutes (the longer the prawns marinate, the more flavor they take in).

In the meantime, add the rice to a lidded saucepan of boiling water. Reduce the heat to a simmer, cover, and cook for 15–20 minutes, or according to the package instructions. Once cooked, drain and rinse under cool water, then spoon the rice into 2 bowls.

Serve the marinated prawns with the rice, along with the carrot, beet, cucumber, scallions, radishes, cilantro, sesame seeds, chili flakes, and a pinch of salt. Pour over any remaining marinade and enjoy cold.

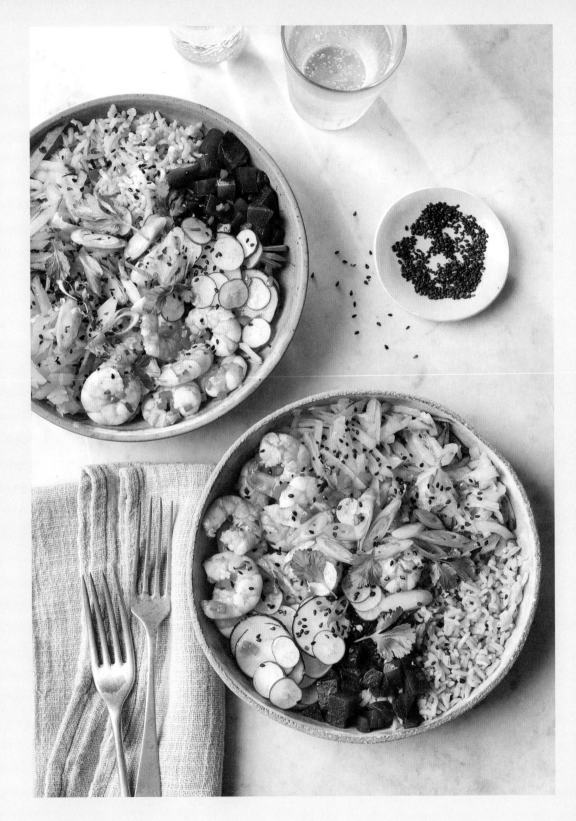

Prawn poke bowl

Spicy lentil vegetable stew

Serves 2
Prep 5 mins
Cook 20 mins

1 tbsp olive oil
½ onion, diced
1 tsp ground cumin
½ tsp cayenne pepper
1 tsp smoked paprika
1 tsp dried thyme
1 garlic clove, finely chopped
1 red pepper, seeded and
   diced
1 carrot, sliced
10 Brussels sprouts, halved
½ broccoli head, cut into
   small florets
7fl oz (200ml) tomato puree,
   ideally from a glass jar
7fl oz (200ml) low-sodium
   vegetable stock
1 tsp tomato paste
juice of ¼ lemon
8 asparagus spears, cut
   into 2in (5cm) pieces
handful of spring greens
2 cups (380g) green lentils,
   drained and rinsed
handful of flat-leaf parsley
   leaves, chopped, to garnish

aids egg and sperm health • supports healthy ovulation • supports early fetal development

Lentils, asparagus, broccoli, and Brussels sprouts make this delicious stew a rich source of folate, supporting egg and sperm quality, ovulation, and early fetal health and development.

Heat the oil in a saucepan over medium heat. Once hot, add the onion and cook for 5 minutes, until soft and translucent.

Add the cumin, cayenne, smoked paprika, thyme, garlic, pepper, carrot, Brussels sprouts, and broccoli. Stir together to coat the vegetables in the spices and cook for 1 minute.

Pour the tomato puree, stock, tomato paste, and lemon juice into the pan. Bring to a boil then reduce the heat and simmer for 15 minutes. Add the asparagus, spring greens, and lentils in the last 5 minutes of the cooking time. Divide the stew between 2 bowls, garnish with the parsley, and serve right away.

Flex it—*For a meat option, add in 9oz (250g) lean beef strips to the pan after cooking the onion and cook for 5 minutes, stirring, until browned, then continue with the recipe.*

Kale, mackerel, *and* pearl barley salad

Serves 2

Prep 5 mins

Cook 15 mins, plus cooling

¼ cup (50g) pearl barley

9fl oz (250ml) low-sodium
  vegetable stock

handful of kale

313.4oz (80g) carton of
  chickpeas, drained and
  rinsed

10 sun-dried tomatoes

2 cooked mackerel fillets,
  flaked

½ avocado, sliced

1 tbsp sunflower seeds

For the dressing

1 tbsp tahini

1 tbsp extra-virgin olive oil

1 tsp white wine vinegar

juice of ¼ lemon

pinch of freshly ground
  black pepper

**may support implantation • helps reduce
inflammation • provides antioxidants**

Whole grain pearl barley promotes uterine health
and implantation. Mackerel adds anti-inflammatory
omega-3s; chickpeas provide plant-based protein;
and kale and tomatoes supply key antioxidants.

Add the pearl barley and stock to a saucepan. Bring
to a boil then reduce the heat and simmer for 10–15
minutes, until the water is absorbed and the pearl
barley has puffed up and softened. Steam the kale
over the pan for a couple of minutes to soften it.
Allow the pearl barley and kale to cool.

In a small bowl, whisk together the dressing
ingredients, adding a splash of cold water for a
looser consistency if desired.

Add the pearl barley to a large serving bowl, along
with the kale, chickpeas, tomatoes, mackerel fillets,
avocado, and sunflower seeds. Pour over the tahini
dressing, toss to combine, and serve right away.

Spicy chicken *with* tabbouleh

Serves 2
Prep 5 mins
Marinate 15–60 mins
Cook 45 mins

**2 chicken breast fillets
    (about 5½oz/150g each)**
½ red onion, cut into wedges
½ cup (70g) bulgur wheat
2 large tomatoes, diced
¼ cucumber, diced
8 black olives
**a large handful of flat-leaf
    parsley leaves, chopped**
**a large handful of mint
    leaves, chopped, plus
    extra to garnish**
1 tbsp pomegranate seeds
juice and zest of ½ lemon
2 tbsp Greek yogurt, to serve

For the marinade
1 tbsp olive oil
1 tsp ground cumin
1 tsp paprika
½ tsp ground coriander
¼ tsp ground cinnamon
juice of ¼ lemon

aids egg and sperm health • may support progesterone levels • may help conception time

Chicken is an excellent source of lean protein, essential for egg and sperm development. The addition of tomatoes, red onions, and pomegranate provides an abundance of vitamin C, thought to support progesterone levels and conception times.

Preheat the oven to 475°F (220°C). Mix the marinade ingredients in a bowl. Add the chicken and onion, cover, and marinate for 15–60 minutes (the longer the chicken marinates, the more flavor it takes in).

Place the marinated chicken and onion in an ovenproof dish and bake for 45 minutes, until the chicken has turned opaque and the juices run clear when pierced with a knife. Let rest for 5 minutes before slicing into ½–¾in (1–2cm) wide strips.

In the meantime, fill a small lidded saucepan with water and bring to a boil. Once boiling, add the bulgur wheat, cover, then reduce the heat and simmer for 15 minutes, or according to the package instructions. Drain and rinse under cold water.

For the tabbouleh, add the tomato, cucumber, olives, parsley, mint, pomegranate seeds, and lemon juice and zest to the pan with the bulgur and stir to combine. Serve the chicken and onion with the tabbouleh and the yogurt on the side.

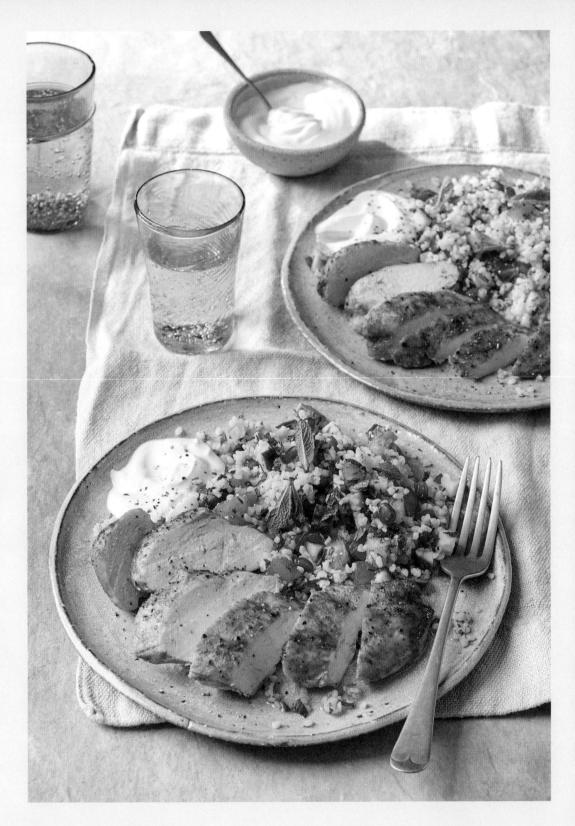

Spicy chicken with tabbouleh

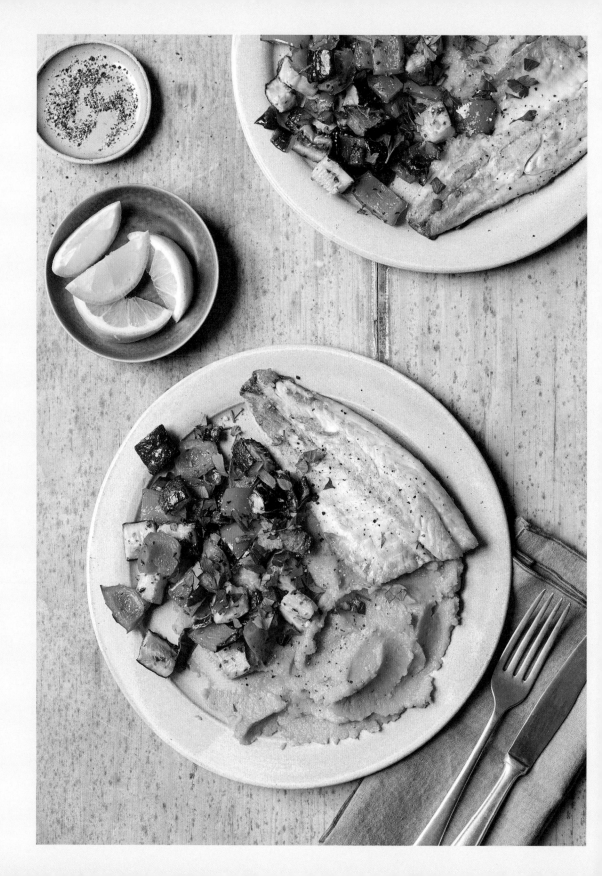

Sea bass *with* roasted vegetables

Serves 2
Prep 5 mins
Cook 25–30 mins

½ **red onion, diced**
1 red pepper, seeded
and chopped
½ **zucchini, diced**
2 tbsp vegetable oil
1 tsp dried oregano
pinch of salt and freshly
ground black pepper
2 sweet potatoes, peeled
and diced
1 tbsp milk or plant-based
alternative
2 sea bass fillets (about
3¼oz/90g each)
handful of flat-leaf parsley,
chopped, to garnish
juice of ¼ lemon, plus
lemon wedges, to serve

may support implantation • provides antioxidants • supports healthy ovulation

This colorful dish is a nutritional powerhouse. Sea bass is high in selenium, supporting egg health and promoting a receptive uterine lining. It also has iodine, key for thyroid health and, in turn, ovulation. A rainbow of veggies add a variety of antioxidants.

Preheat the oven to 425°F (200°C). Put the onion, red pepper, and zucchini in a baking dish. Add 1 tablespoon of the oil and the oregano, season, and toss. Roast for 25–30 minutes, until the veggies are soft. In the meantime, put the sweet potato in a saucepan of boiling water. Cook for 20 minutes, until soft. Drain, add the milk, and mash until smooth.

In the last 5 minutes of the vegetable cooking time, heat the remaining oil in a skillet over medium-high heat. Score the skin side of the fish to prevent it from shrinking when cooking. Place the sea bass fillets in the pan, skin-side down, and press down on the fish to prevent it from curling. Fry for 4 minutes, then flip the fillets over and cook for another minute.

Remove the vegetables from the oven, garnish them with the parsley, pour over the lemon juice, and toss to combine. Serve the sea bass with the roasted vegetables, sweet potato mash, and lemon wedges.

Salmon *with* watercress sauce *and* Puy lentils

Serves 2
Prep 5 mins
Cook 25 mins

²/₃ cup (120g) Puy lentils
11fl oz (320ml) low-sodium
    vegetable stock
handful of asparagus
handful of broccolini
handful of kale
1 tsp white wine vinegar
1 tbsp olive oil
2 salmon fillets
freshly ground black pepper
6 walnuts, crushed
lemon wedges, to serve

For the watercress sauce
2¹/₃ cup (80g) watercress
3¹/₂oz (100g) crème fraîche
juice of ¹/₄ lemon
¹/₄ tsp Dijon mustard

has anti-inflammatory properties • aids egg and sperm health • may help support implantation

Essential omega-3s, abundant in salmon and walnuts, are a key component of a fertility diet, reducing harmful inflammation, supporting egg and sperm health, and aiding implantation. Lentils, kale, and broccolini add fiber and folate.

Place the Puy lentils in a saucepan and cover with the stock. Bring to a boil, then reduce the heat and simmer for 20–25 minutes. In the last 5 minutes, steam the asparagus, broccolini, and kale over the lentil pan. When cooked, drain any excess liquid from the lentils then stir in the white wine vinegar.

Halfway through the lentil cooking time, heat the oil in a skillet over medium heat. Once hot, add the salmon fillets, skin-side down, and cook for 10 minutes, turning halfway through, until just opaque and the flesh flakes easily with a fork.

To make the watercress sauce, place all the ingredients in a food processor and pulse to a smooth consistency. If desired, gently heat the watercress sauce in a saucepan. Spoon the lentils onto 2 plates, top with the salmon fillets, drizzle over the watercress sauce, and add a crack of black pepper. Sprinkle the walnuts over the lentils. Serve the salmon and lentils alongside the vegetables, with lemon wedges on the side.

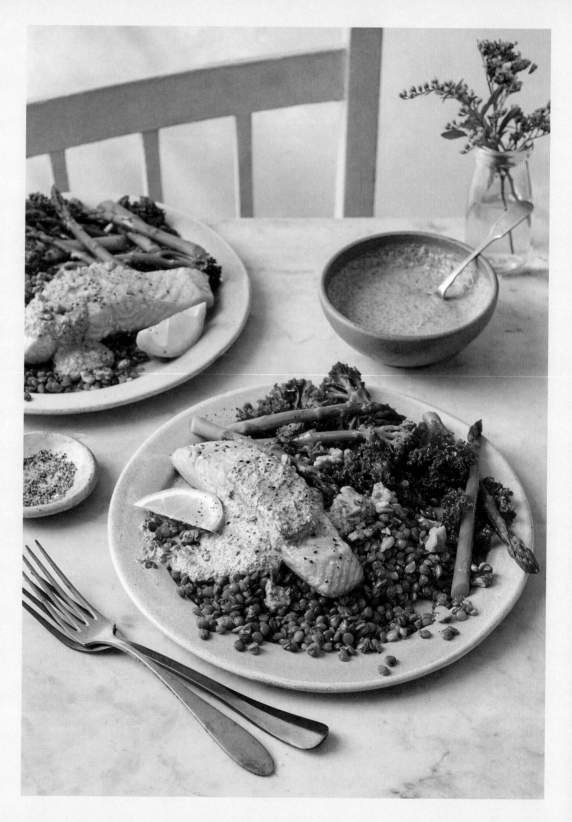

Salmon with watercress sauce and Puy lentils

157

Butternut squash tarka dhal

Serves 2
Prep 5 mins
Cook 30 mins

½ butternut squash, peeled
and diced
2 tbsp olive oil
1 tbsp ground cumin
¾ cup (150g) dried red lentils,
rinsed
1 tsp turmeric
12fl oz (350ml) low-sodium
vegetable stock
7fl oz (200ml) reduced-fat
coconut milk
1 tsp tomato paste
1 tsp cumin seeds
1 tsp mustard seeds
1 tsp coriander seeds
½ onion, thinly sliced
handful of Brussels sprouts,
thinly sliced
1 garlic clove, crushed
¼ tsp cayenne pepper
¼ tsp ground cinnamon
1in (2.5cm) piece of ginger,
peeled and finely chopped
1 tsp garam masala
handful of cilantro leaves,
to garnish
1 tbsp sesame seeds,
to garnish

provides antioxidants • aids egg and sperm health

Squash is rich in antioxidants, including beta-carotene and vitamins C and E, supporting overall fertility for women and men. The variety of herbs and spices adds to the antioxidant content.

Preheat the oven to 425°F (200°C). Place the squash in an ovenproof dish, drizzle over 1 tablespoon of the oil, add the cumin, and toss to combine. Roast for 30 minutes. Put the lentils, turmeric, and stock in a saucepan and bring to a boil. Reduce the heat and simmer for 20–25 minutes. Add the coconut milk and tomato paste in the last 10 minutes.

In the meantime, place the cumin seeds, mustard seeds, and coriander seeds in a small skillet. Dry-fry for 2–3 minutes, stirring, until they pop and release their aromas. Grind the spices in a pestle and mortar to a powder.

For the tarka, heat the remaining oil in a large skillet over medium heat. Add the ground spices, onion, and sprouts and cook for 10 minutes. Add the garlic, cayenne, cinnamon, ginger, and garam masala. Cook for 5 minutes, stirring often. Mash the squash into the lentil pan and spoon into 2 bowls. Add the tarka and garnish with the cilantro and sesame seeds. If batch cooking, keep covered in the fridge for up to 3 days, or freeze in an airtight container for up to 6 months.

Spicy prawn skewers
with mango salad

Serves 2
Prep 5 mins
Marinate 10–20 mins
Cook 20 mins

1 tsp paprika
1 tsp lemon juice
1 tsp reduced-salt soy sauce
2 tbsp olive oil
1 tsp ground cumin
1 garlic clove, finely chopped
1 tsp dried thyme
8¹/₂oz (240g) raw king prawns,
**   peeled and deveined**
2¹/₂oz (70g) quinoa, drained
**   and rinsed under cold water**

For the mango salad
¹/₂ mango, diced
¹/₂ red onion, thinly sliced
¹/₂ tsp chili flakes
juice of 1 lime
handful of cilantro leaves,
**   chopped**
handful of arugula
1 tsp extra-virgin olive oil
¹/₂ avocado, pitted and sliced
1 tsp sesame seeds, toasted

supports weight management • helps reduce inflammation • provides antioxidants

An excellent source of protein and essential omega-3s, prawns are also low in calories, making this satisfying dish a good choice for weight control. Bright mangoes and red onion add antioxidant vitamin C, to help support progesterone levels.

If using wooden skewers, presoak these in a bowl of water before cooking. In a small bowl, mix together the paprika, lemon juice, soy sauce, 1 tablespoon of the olive oil, cumin, garlic, and thyme. Add the prawns to the bowl and coat in the mixture. Set aside to marinate for 10–20 minutes.

In the meantime, place the quinoa in a lidded saucepan with 14fl oz (400ml) of water. Bring to a boil, then reduce the heat to a simmer. Cover and cook for 10–15 minutes, or according to the package instructions, until the quinoa has softened and the liquid has been absorbed. Set aside.

To make the mango salad, combine all the ingredients together in a bowl.

Heat the remaining oil in a skillet. Skewer the prawns and cook for 2 minutes on each side. Serve the skewers together with the quinoa and mango salad.

(photographed overleaf)

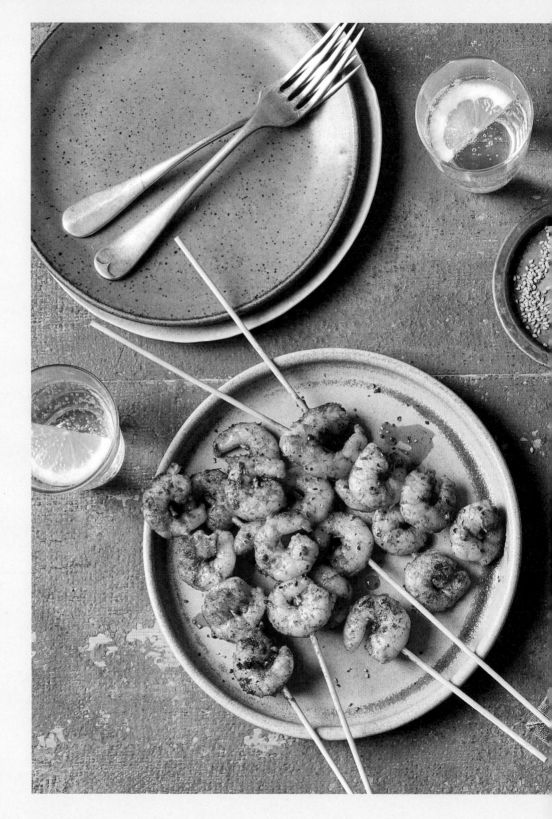

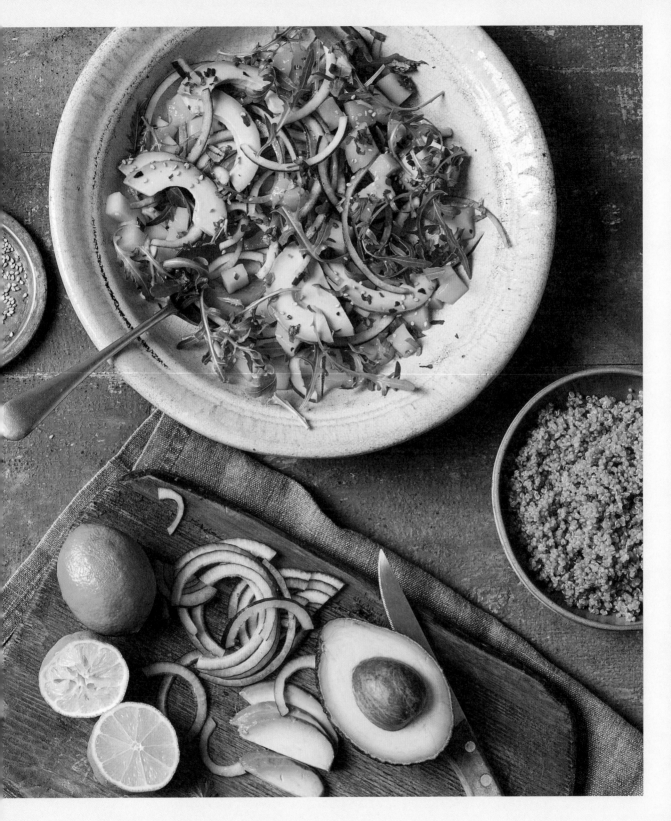

Spicy prawn skewers with mango salad

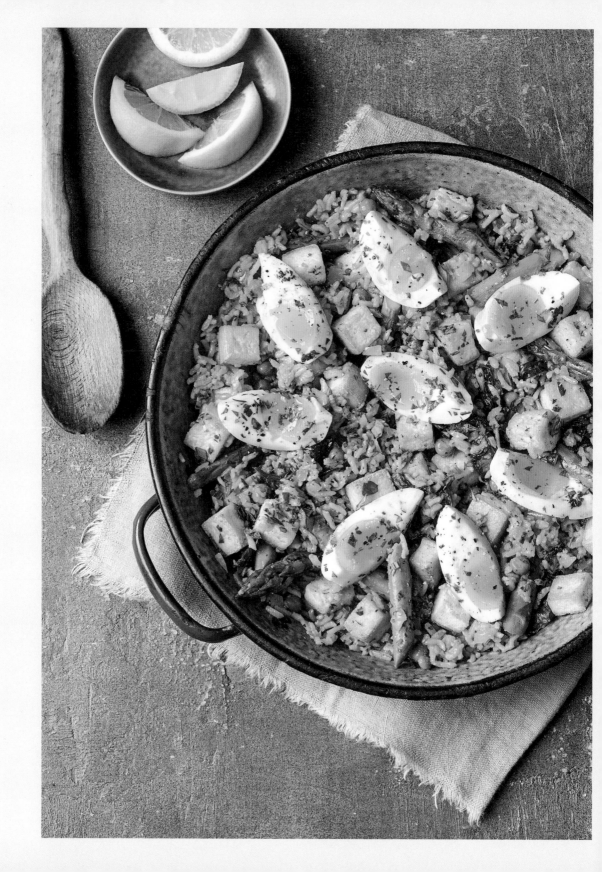

Smoked tofu kedgeree

Serves 2
Prep 5 mins
Cook 30 mins

1 tbsp olive oil
1 block extra-firm smoked
   tofu, drained and diced
$^1/_2$ onion, finely chopped
1 garlic clove, finely
   chopped
$^1/_4$ tsp cayenne pepper
1 tbsp curry powder
1 tsp garam masala
$^1/_2$ tsp turmeric
$^3/_4$ cup (150g) brown rice
10fl oz (300ml) low-sodium
   vegetable stock
2 eggs
4 tbsp garden peas, fresh
   or frozen
handful of asparagus, cut
   into 2in (5cm) pieces
handful of spinach
lemon wedges, to serve
handful of flat-leaf parsley,
   to garnish

supplies fiber • may help reduce conception time

This gently spiced veggie kedgeree provides high-quality plant-based protein as well as iron and selenium from the tofu. Eggs supply the fertility-supporting nutrients choline and iodine.

Heat the oil in a lidded saucepan over medium heat. Once hot, add the tofu and fry on each side until lightly browned. Remove from the pan and set aside.

Add the onion to the pan and cook for about 5 minutes, until softened. Add the garlic and cook for 1 minute. Add the cayenne, curry powder, garam masala, and turmeric and cook for a further 2 minutes. Add the rice and stir to coat it in the spice mixture, then add the stock. Bring to a simmer, cover, and cook for 15–20 minutes, until the rice is tender and has absorbed the stock.

In the meantime, boil the eggs (6 minutes for soft-boiled, 7 minutes for hard-boiled) and cook the peas in boiling water for 1–2 minutes. Cool the eggs under cold water then peel and quarter them. In the last 5 minutes of the rice cooking time, add the asparagus and spinach to the rice pan to soften slightly. Once the rice is cooked, add the peas and tofu. Stir them through the rice to heat them through. Top with the boiled eggs and serve with lemon wedges and a garnish of parsley.

Spinach *and* ricotta chicken *with* a warm lima bean salad

Serves 2
Prep 10 mins
Cook 30 mins

1 tbsp olive oil
1 tsp paprika
1 garlic clove, finely chopped
2 chicken breasts, about
    5¹/₂oz (150g) each
4 handfuls of spinach
2 tbsp ricotta
10 green olives, pitted
    and halved

For the lima bean salad
1 tsp olive oil
handful of broccolini
¹/₂ x 13.4oz (380g) carton
    of lima beans, drained
    and rinsed
1 tsp lemon juice
1 tsp pesto, plus extra
    to serve, if desired
1 tsp mixed seeds
handful of basil leaves,
    to garnish

may help regulate menstrual cycle • supports early fetal development

This satisfying chicken dish delivers iron, key for a healthy menstrual cycle, and vitamin B12, low levels of which are linked to fertility issues. In addition, spinach supplies folate, supporting both menstruation and early fetal development.

Preheat the oven to 400°F (190°C). Place the oil, paprika, and garlic in a small bowl and stir to combine. Rub the oil mixture evenly over both sides of the chicken. Use a sharp knife to cut an opening into one side of each chicken breast.

Wilt the spinach over a saucepan of boiling water, then drain excess liquid. Place the spinach in a bowl with the ricotta and olives and combine. Spoon the mixture into the chicken breast incisions. Place the chicken on a baking sheet and bake for 25–30 minutes, until opaque and juices run clear when the chicken is cut with a knife.

Ten minutes before the chicken is ready, make the salad. Heat the olive oil in a small skillet over medium heat. Once hot, add the broccolini and cook for 5 minutes. Add the lima beans, lemon juice, pesto, and seeds, and cook for another 2 minutes. Spoon the warm salad onto 2 plates and garnish with the basil. Serve the salad alongside the chicken, drizzling some extra pesto over the chicken if desired.

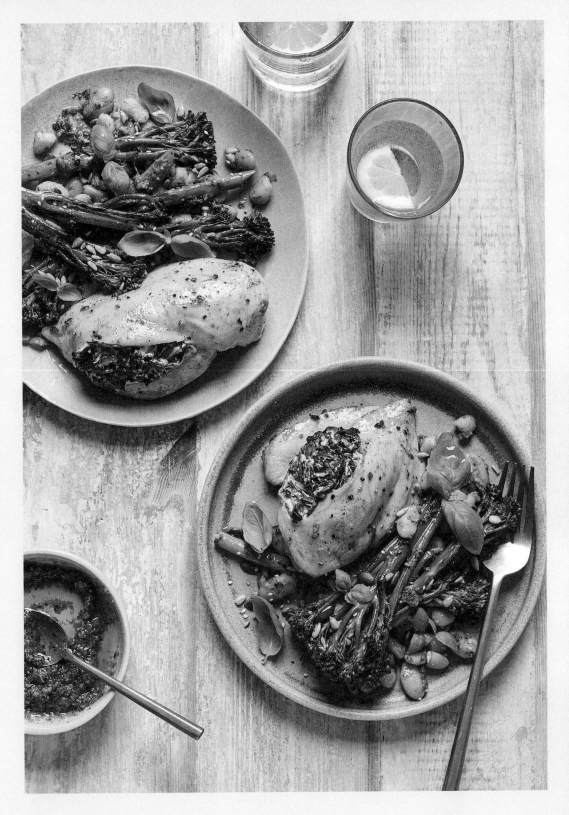

Spinach and ricotta chicken with a warm lima bean salad   165

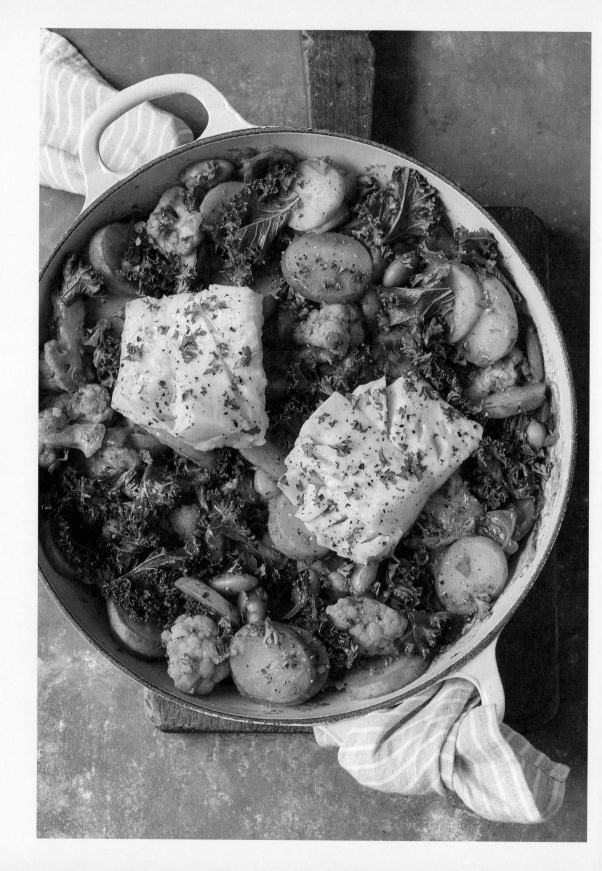

One-pot smoky fish

Serves 2
Prep 5 mins
Cook 35 mins

1 tbsp olive oil
¹/₂ red onion, diced
8 new potatoes, sliced
1 garlic clove, crushed
1 tsp smoked paprika
¹/₂ tsp cayenne pepper
13.4oz (380g) carton of lima beans, drained and rinsed
juice of ¹/₂ lemon
¹/₂ cauliflower, cut into small florets
3¹/₂fl oz (100ml) tomato puree, ideally from a glass jar
12 cherry tomatoes, halved
1 bay leaf
7fl oz (200ml) fish stock, ideally reduced sodium
2 handfuls of curly kale
2 fillets of cod or haddock (about 5¹/₂oz/150g each)
handful of curly parsley, chopped, to garnish

promotes hormonal balance • supports early pregnancy • aids egg and sperm health

White fish such as cod or haddock provide lean protein. They also supply vitamin B6, which supports progesterone levels; B12, which promotes healthy sperm and is linked to a reduced miscarriage risk; and iodine, a key fertility nutrient.

Heat the oil in a lidded saucepan over medium heat. Once hot, add the onion and potatoes, cover, and cook for 5 minutes. Add the garlic, paprika, and cayenne, then cook for another 2 minutes.

Add the lima beans, lemon juice, cauliflower, tomato puree, tomatoes, bay leaf, and the stock. Cover the pan and simmer for 20 minutes, until the potatoes are just cooked and can be pierced easily with a knife.

Add the kale and stir this through. Place the fish on top of the stew, reduce the heat to low, cover, and cook for about 8 minutes, stirring gently once or twice, until the fish is cooked and flakes easily with a knife. Remove the bay leaf. Sprinkle on the parsley to serve.

If batch cooking, store in an airtight container in the fridge for up to 3 days, or freeze the sauce without the fish in an airtight container for up to 3 months.

Chicken *and* rice casserole

Serves 2
Prep 5 mins
Cook 35 mins

1 red pepper, seeded and
   sliced
1 red onion, cut into wedges
12 button mushrooms, halved
12 cherry tomatoes, halved
pinch of salt and freshly
   ground black pepper
1 tsp balsamic vinegar
1 tbsp olive oil
2 chicken breast fillets
   (about 5½oz/150g each)
²/₃ cup (100g) whole grain or
   wild rice
1 tbsp pesto
13.4oz (380g) carton of black
   beans, drained and rinsed
handful of basil leaves, torn,
   to garnish
juice of ¼ lemon
handful of arugula, to serve

Flex it—*For a veggie swap,
omit the chicken and add 2oz (60g)
sliced Halloumi cheese. Arrange it
on top of the roasted vegetables,
then place under a medium–high
grill for 5 minutes.*

aids egg and sperm health • may help support implantation

This flavorsome dish has protein, healthy fats, fueling carbs, and fiber, keeping you going between meals. Mushrooms and chicken have the antioxidant mineral selenium, which promotes egg and sperm health, while whole grain rice may support implantation.

Preheat the oven to 425°F (200°C). Place the red pepper, onion, mushrooms, and tomatoes in a large ovenproof dish, season, and drizzle with the balsamic vinegar and olive oil. Place the chicken breasts on top of the vegetables and roast in the oven for 25–30 minutes, until the chicken is cooked through and the vegetables are softened and golden.

In the meantime, add the rice to a lidded saucepan of boiling water. Reduce the heat to a simmer, cover, and cook according to the package instructions.

Remove the chicken from the vegetables and cut into thick slices. Add the rice, pesto, and black beans to the vegetables and stir together. Arrange the chicken slices on top. Garnish with the basil leaves and pour over the lemon juice. Serve with a side of arugula.

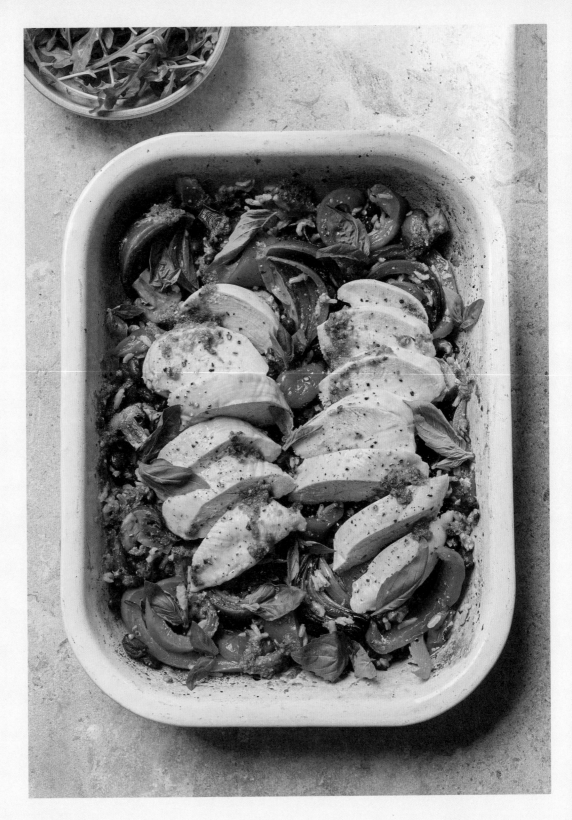

Chicken and rice casserole

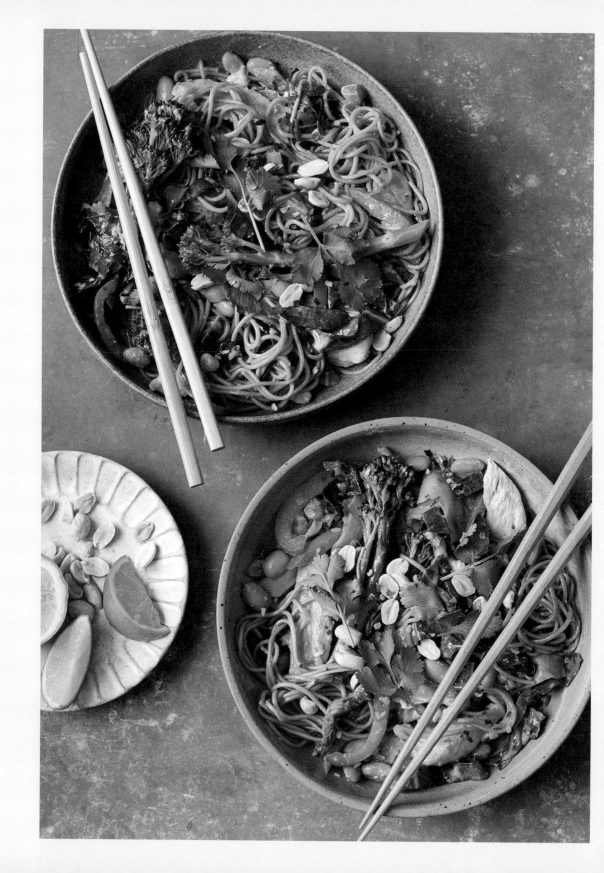

Chicken *and* vegetable stir-fry *with* noodles

Serves 2
Prep 5–10 mins
Cook 15 mins

2 whole wheat noodle nests
   or soba noodles
1 tbsp vegetable oil
2 chicken breasts (about 5½oz/
   150g each), cut into strips
½ tsp crushed chili
2.5cm (1in) piece of ginger, diced
1 garlic clove, diced
1 scallion, sliced
½ red pepper, seeded and
   cut into strips
handful of broccolini
1 carrot, cut into ribbon strips
handful of spring greens, chopped
handful of edamame beans
1 egg
handful of cilantro leaves,
   chopped
1 tbsp unsalted peanuts
½ tsp chili flakes
lime wedges, to serve

For the peanut sauce
1 tbsp low-sodium soy sauce
1 tbsp unsalted smooth
   peanut butter
1 tsp rice wine vinegar
1 tsp lime juice

aids egg and sperm quality • provides antioxidants

This tasty dish is packed with protein, fiber, and fertility-promoting antioxidants such as selenium, supporting egg maturation and sperm production. Peanut butter adds healthy fats and vitamin E.

Mix together the peanut sauce ingredients and set aside. Add the noodles to a saucepan of boiling water and cook for 10 minutes, or according to the packet instructions. Drain the noodles and set aside.

In the meantime, heat the oil in a skillet or wok over medium heat. Once hot, add the chicken and cook for 10 minutes, until opaque and the juices run clear when pierced with a knife. Add the crushed chili, ginger, garlic, scallion, red pepper, broccolini, carrot, spring greens, and edamame beans and fry for 5 minutes.

Remove the pan from the heat. Make a small space in the ingredients and crack an egg gently into this. Scramble the egg with a wooden spoon then mix it in with the rest of the ingredients. Add the noodles and toss. Add the peanut sauce, top with the cilantro, peanuts, and chili flakes, and serve with lime wedges.

Flex it—*Swap the chicken for 1 block of extra-firm tofu. Drain and rinse the tofu then dice it. Fry it in the oil 2–3 minutes each side, then add to the pan with the veggies to heat through.*

Burrito bowl

Serves 4
Prep 5–10 mins
Cook 35–40 mins

1 tbsp vegetable oil
½ small onion, diced
1 garlic clove, diced
9oz (250g) lean ground beef
1 red pepper, seeded
   and diced
¼ tsp chili powder
1 tsp ground cumin
1 tsp smoked paprika
½ tsp ground cinnamon
3½fl oz (100ml) tomato puree,
   ideally from a glass jar
12 cherry tomatoes, halved
1 bay leaf
13.4oz (380g) carton of kidney
   beans, drained and rinsed
½ cup (100g) brown rice
juice of ½ lime

To serve
4 romaine lettuce leaves,
   roughly chopped
1 avocado, mashed
2 tbsp corn
2 tbsp yogurt
handful of cilantro leaves
lime wedges

aids egg and sperm health • promotes hormonal balance • may support implantation

This high-protein bowl supports tissue renewal for healthy sperm and eggs. Beef also provides vitamin B12, zinc, selenium, and iron. Whole grain rice steadies blood sugars, insulin, and other hormones and promotes a healthy uterine lining for implantation.

Heat the oil in a large saucepan over medium heat. Once hot, add the onion. Fry, stirring frequently, for 5 minutes, until soft and translucent. Add the garlic and cook for another minute. Add the ground beef and cook for 5–10 minutes, until browned. Add the red pepper, chili powder, cumin, paprika, and cinnamon, stir to coat the vegetables in the spices, and cook for 2 minutes. Add the tomato puree, tomatoes, and bay leaf. Bring to a simmer and cook for 15–20 minutes. In the last 5 minutes, add the kidney beans.

In the meantime, add the rice to a lidded saucepan with 7fl oz (200ml) boiling water. Reduce to a simmer, cover, and cook according to the package instructions. Remove from the heat, add the lime juice, and stir. Spoon the rice into 2 bowls with the chili (remove the bay leaf). Serve with the lettuce, avocado, corn, yogurt, cilantro, and lime wedges. If batch cooking the chili, keep the remainder covered in the fridge for up to 3 days. Or freeze in an airtight container for up to 3 months.

Flex it—*For a vegetarian bowl, simply remove the ground beef.*

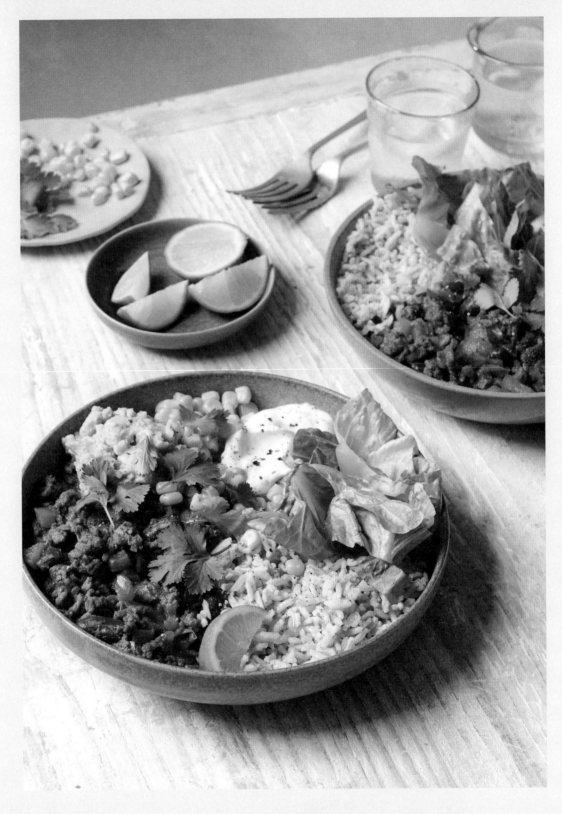

Burrito bowl

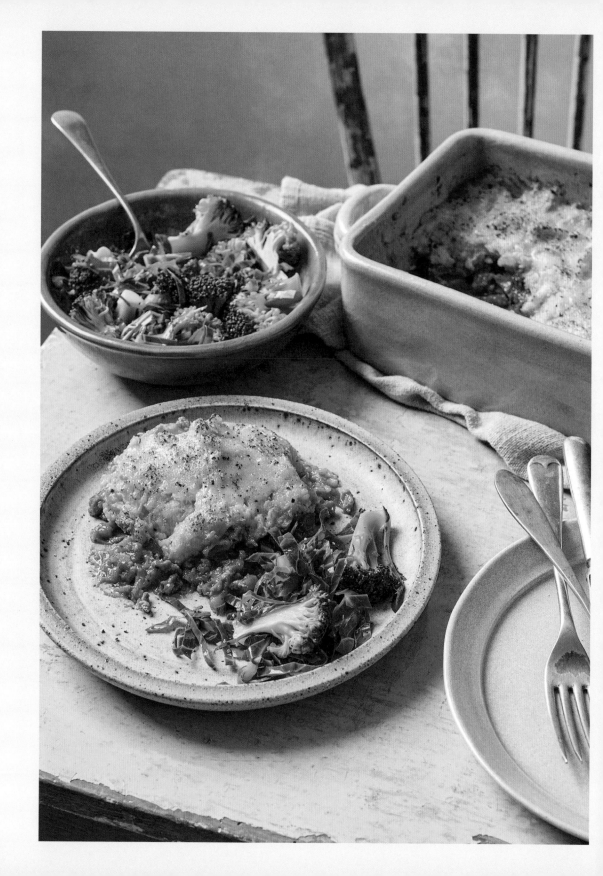

Sweet potato cottage pie

Serves 2
Prep 5 mins
Cook 60 mins

**2 sweet potatoes, peeled
and diced**
**1 tbsp milk or plant-based
alternative**
1 tbsp olive oil
½ onion, diced
1 celery stalk, diced
1 large carrot, diced
1 garlic clove, finely chopped
1 tbsp dried thyme
9oz (250g) lean ground beef
**pinch of salt and freshly
ground black pepper**
**14fl oz (400ml) tomato puree,
ideally from a glass jar**
**7fl oz (200ml) reduced-fat
beef stock**
**1oz (30g) Cheddar cheese,
grated**
**handful of broccoli, cut
into small florets**
**handful of spring greens,
finely chopped**

Flex it—*For a vegetarian option,
swap the ground beef for a 13.4oz
(380g) carton of green lentils.*

supplies fiber • promotes hormonal balance

Swapping in sweet potatoes in this classic dish
ups your fiber intake and provides a lower glycemic
index, helping steady blood sugars, insulin, and
other hormones. Beef also provides vitamin B12,
selenium, zinc, and iron.

Preheat the oven to 400°F (180°C). Add the sweet
potatoes to a saucepan of boiling water and cook
for 20 minutes, until soft, then drain. Add the milk
and mash the potatoes to a creamy consistency.

In the meantime, heat the oil in a skillet over medium
heat. Once hot, add the onion, celery, carrot, garlic,
and thyme and fry for 5 minutes. Add the ground beef,
season, and fry for another 5 minutes, until browned.
Pour in the tomato puree and stock and simmer for
10 minutes.

Pour the beef mixture into the bottom of a baking dish,
spoon the sweet potato mash on top, and sprinkle with
the cheese. Place in the oven for 30–40 minutes.

Five minutes before serving, steam the broccoli and
spring greens. Serve the pie with the steamed green
vegetables, adding a crack of black pepper if desired.
If batch cooking, keep covered in the fridge for up to
3 days or store in an airtight container in the freezer
for up to 2 months.

Savory snacks

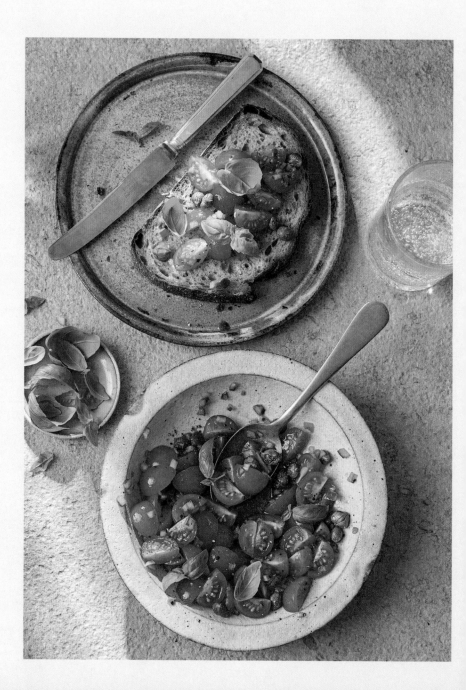

Enjoy this appetizing selection of savory bites, perfect for a quick snack, nibbles, or starters.

Ideally, the energy your main meals provide keeps you going from one meal to the next. Inevitably, though, there are days when energy levels drop and you crave an extra "something." Often, when tempted to snack, people reach for something sugary and processed. Having these tasty, nutrient-dense savory treats on hand is just the ticket to nip hunger pangs in the bud and avoid energy-sapping sugar spikes.

From creamy pâtés and dips to favorites such as muffins, falafels, bruschetta, and crostini, these delicious bites provide a compact package of fertility-promoting nutrients, supporting your fertility diet throughout the week.

Mackerel pâté

helps reduce inflammation • aids egg and sperm health • may support implantation

Creamy and delicious, this pâté delivers anti-inflammatory omega-3s in mackerel, supporting egg and sperm health. Beets add dietary nitrates, which enhance blood flow to the uterus. Both omega-3s and nitrates promote a healthy uterine lining, increasing the chances of successful implantation.

Serves 2
Prep 5 mins
Cook 5 mins

2 mackerel fillets, about 5–7oz/ 140–200g combined weight, cooked and flaked, or 4.4oz (125g) can of mackerel in olive oil or spring water (drained weight about 3oz/90g), flaked

1 tbsp cream cheese
1 tsp paprika
pinch of freshly ground black pepper
handful of flat-leaf parsley leaves, chopped
2 slices of whole wheat sourdough bread
2 pickled beets, sliced
1 celery stalk, thinly sliced

Add the mackerel to a bowl with the cream cheese, paprika, black pepper, and parsley and mix thoroughly with a fork.

Lightly toast the bread. Spread the mackerel pâté on the toast and top with the slices of pickled beets and celery. Store leftover pâté, covered, in the fridge for up to 3 days.

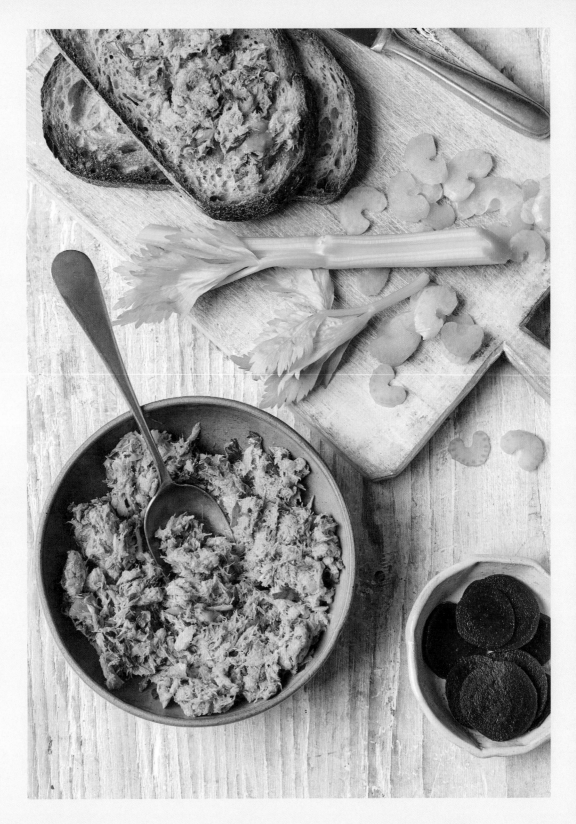

Mackerel pâté

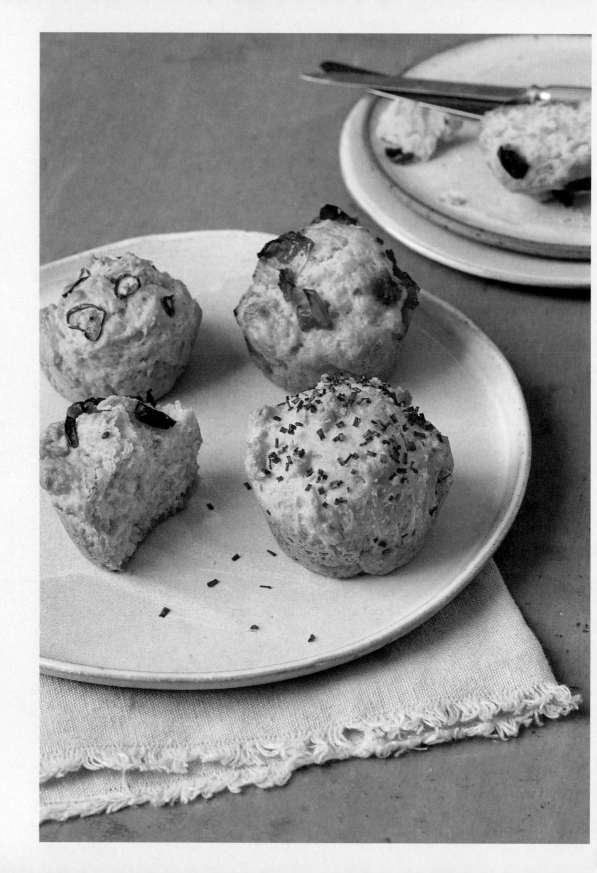

Savory muffins

Makes 4
Prep 5 mins
Cook 25 mins

¾ cup (100g) self-rising flour
½ tsp baking powder
1 egg
3½fl oz (100ml) milk or
   plant-based alternative
1⅓ tbsp(20g) yogurt
1½ tbsp vegetable oil
1 garlic clove, diced

Extras (choose 1): 4 sun-dried
   tomatoes, diced; handful
   of fresh chives, chopped;
   4 olives, diced; 3 jalapeño
   peppers, halved; 1 scallion,
   diced; 1½oz (40g) feta
   cheese, crumbled

supports ovulatory health • aids sperm health

Add your flavor of choice to these crave-worthy muffins. Using vegetable oil provides healthy fats as well as vitamin E, while the dairy content provides protein and vitamin B12, supporting ovulation and sperm health.

Preheat the oven to 400°F (180°C). Grease 4 cups in a muffin pan.

Place the flour and baking powder in a bowl. Place the egg, milk, yogurt, oil, and garlic in a separate bowl and mix these together. Pour the wet ingredients into the flour and baking powder, then fold in your additional ingredient of choice.

Divide the mixture between the 4 muffin cups and bake in the oven for 25 minutes. Enjoy warm or cooled. The muffins can be stored in an airtight container in the fridge for up to 3 days.

Hummus *with* olives *and* toasted pine nuts

Serves 2–4
Prep 5 mins
Cook 5 mins

1 tbsp pine nuts
13.4oz (380g) carton of chickpeas (drained weight 8oz/230g)
2 tbsp extra-virgin olive oil, divided
juice of ½ lemon
1 garlic clove, finely chopped
1 tbsp tahini
½ tsp ground cumin
¼ tsp ground coriander
handful of olives, halved
pinch of smoked paprika
vegetable crudités of choice, to serve

supports healthy ovulation • promotes hormonal balance • aids sperm health

Effortless to whip up, this homemade hummus wins on flavor. Chickpeas supply iron and plant-based protein, thought to be especially helpful for ovulation. Tahini adds selenium, a strong antioxidant that supports egg and sperm health.

Toast the pine nuts in a skillet over medium heat for 2–3 minutes, stirring constantly, until just turning golden.

To make the hummus, place the chickpeas, 1 tablespoon of the olive oil, the lemon juice, garlic, tahini, cumin, and coriander in a food processor and pulse to form a creamy consistency. Add a splash of water if it becomes too thick.

Spoon the hummus into a bowl and drizzle with the remaining olive oil. Top with the toasted pine nuts, olives, and smoked paprika and serve with vegetable crudités of your choice. Any leftover hummus can be stored in the fridge for up to 3 days.

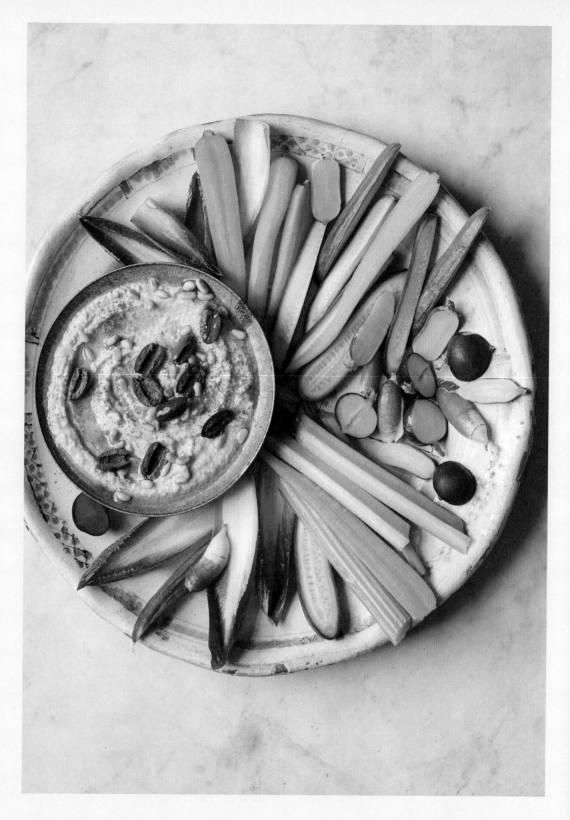

Hummus with olives and toasted pine nuts

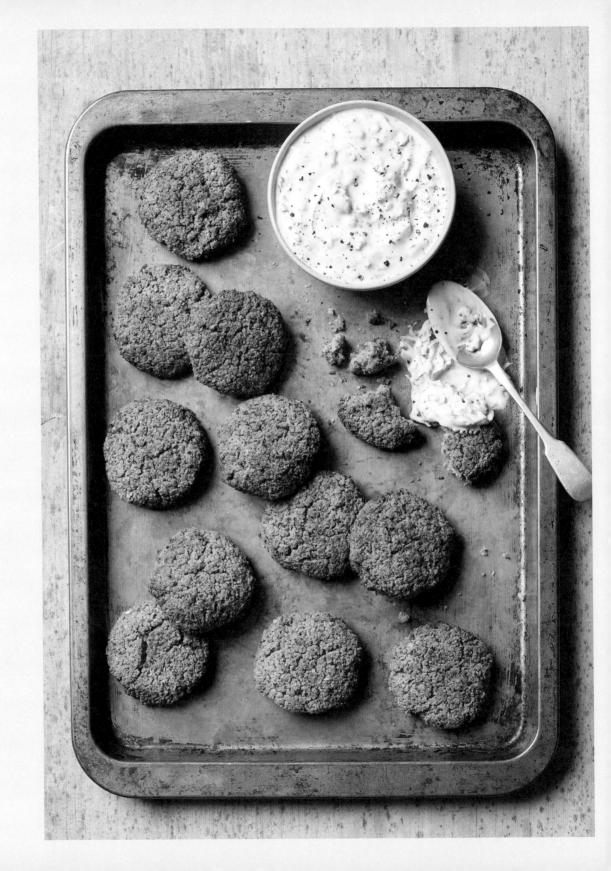

Baked falafel *and* tzatziki

Makes 12
Prep overnight, 8+ hours
Cook 25–30 mins

**2 tbsp extra-virgin olive oil,
    divided**
**³/₄ cup (175g) dried chickpeas,
    soaked in water overnight,
    drained,
    and patted dry**
¹/₂ red onion, diced
1 garlic clove, diced
1 tbsp ground cumin
¹/₂ tsp ground coriander
**pinch of salt and freshly
    ground black pepper**
**handful of cilantro leaves,
    chopped**
**handful of flat-leaf parsley
    leaves, chopped**

For the tzatziki
9oz (250g) Greek yogurt
¹/₂ cucumber, grated
1 tbsp extra-virgin olive oil
1 tsp dried dill
**handful of mint leaves,
    chopped**
1 tsp lemon juice
1 garlic clove, diced
**crack of freshly ground black
    pepper, to serve (optional)**

supports ovulatory health • aids sperm health

With iron and high-quality plant-based protein, chickpeas promote healthy ovulation. Yogurt adds vitamin B12 for sperm health.

Preheat the oven to 425°F (200°C). Pour 1 tablespoon of the olive oil into a baking sheet and heat in the oven while preparing the falafels. Place the chickpeas, the remaining olive oil, red onion, garlic, cumin, coriander, seasoning, cilantro, and parsley in a food processor and pulse until it forms a smooth consistency.

Use your hands to shape the mixture into patties— 2in (5cm) wide and ½in (1cm) thick. Place the patties on the preheated baking sheet and bake for 25–30 minutes, flipping them over in the last 10 minutes so they are lightly browned on both sides.

In the meantime, make the tzatziki by combining all the ingredients in a small bowl and mixing together. Add a crack of black pepper if desired. Serve the falafels with the tzatziki dip.

Store leftover falafels in the fridge in an airtight container for 3–4 days, and store any leftover tzatziki, covered, in the fridge for up to 4 days.

Edamame *and* sesame bowl

supplies folate • may support fertility treatments

This vegan snack is rich in fertility-supporting folate
and plant-based protein from the soy-derived edamame
beans. Soy has been linked to more favorable outcomes
for couples receiving IVF.

Serves 2
Prep 5 mins
Cook 5 mins

**1 cup (160g) shelled edamame
beans
1 tsp extra-virgin olive oil
juice of ¼ lime
1 tbsp sesame seeds
½ tsp chili flakes**

Place the edamame beans in a saucepan of boiling water and cook
for 5 minutes. Drain then rinse the beans under cold water to cool.

Transfer the beans to a bowl. Mix in the olive oil, lime juice, sesame
seeds, and chili flakes before serving.

Tomato *and* basil bruschetta

provides antioxidants • has anti-inflammatory properties • aids sperm health

A staple of the Mediterranean diet, sweet and tangy tomatoes provide key antioxidants such as vitamin C and beta-carotene, helping limit damaging inflammation and in turn support reproductive health. They also supply lycopene, thought to support a good sperm concentration and sperm health.

Serves 2
Prep 15 mins
Marinate 5 mins

12 cherry tomatoes, quartered
$\frac{1}{4}$ red onion, finely chopped
1 tbsp extra-virgin olive oil
1 tsp balsamic vinegar
1 tbsp capers
juice of $\frac{1}{2}$ lemon
$\frac{1}{4}$ tsp chili flakes
2 slices of whole grain bread
handful of basil leaves, chopped, to garnish

Place the tomatoes, red onion, olive oil, balsamic vinegar, capers, lemon juice, and chili flakes in a small bowl and stir to combine. Set aside for 5 minutes to allow the tomatoes to marinate.

Lightly toast the bread. Transfer the tomato mixture onto the toast, leaving most of the liquid in the bowl. Garnish with the basil leaves and enjoy right away.

(photographed overleaf)

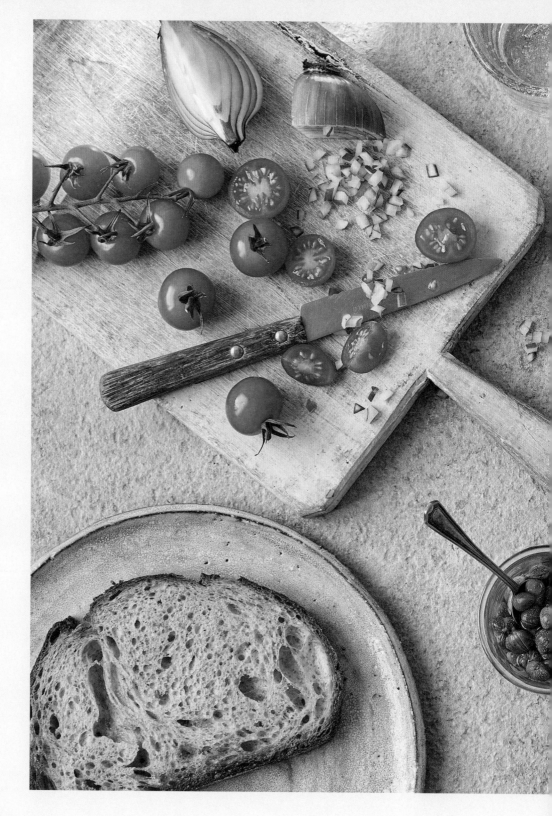

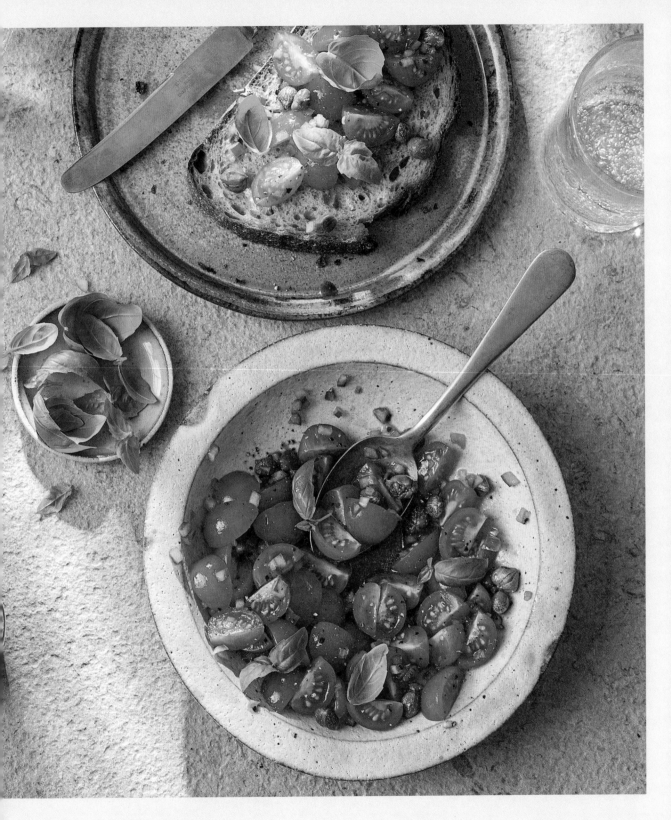

Tomato and basil bruschetta

189

Cannellini bean *and* sun-dried tomato crostini

Serves 4
Prep 5 mins
Cook 10 mins, plus cooling

2 tbsp olive oil, divided
1 shallot, diced
1 garlic clove, crushed
13.4oz (380g) carton of
   cannellini beans, drained
   and rinsed
3¹/₂ tbsp low-sodium
   vegetable stock
¹/₂ tsp dried thyme
juice of ¹/₄ lemon
2–4 slices of whole wheat
   bread, or multigrain
   crispbreads
10 sun-dried tomatoes, diced
handful of flat-leaf parsley,
   to serve

supplies fiber • promotes hormonal balance • provides antioxidants • aids sperm health

Creamy cannellini beans and whole wheat toast mean this tasty snack delivers on fiber, to support gut health and keep blood sugars, insulin, and hormones in check. Intensely sweet sun-dried tomatoes add antioxidants, including lycopene for healthy sperm.

Heat 1 tablespoon of the olive oil in a small saucepan over medium heat. Once hot, add the shallot and cook for 5 minutes, until softened. Add the garlic, cannellini beans, stock, thyme, and lemon juice, and simmer for 5 minutes. Set aside to cool a little.

Gently mash the slightly cooled bean mixture to make a rough but spreadable consistency. Enjoy warm or cool further (it will thicken as it cools). If using bread, lightly toast the bread, then top the toast or crispbreads with the bean mixture. Drizzle remaining olive oil on top and add the sun-dried tomatoes and a garnish of parsley to serve. Any excess bean mixture can be stored, covered, in the fridge for 3–4 days.

190

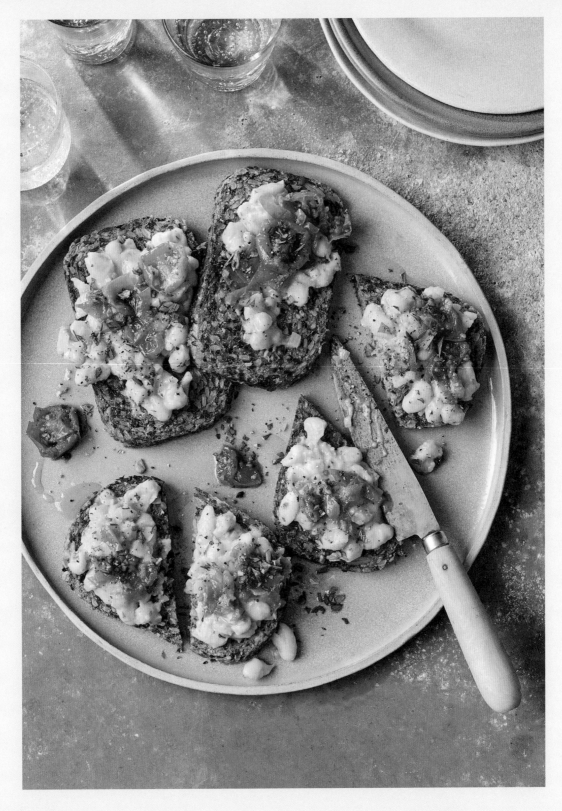

Cannellini bean and sun-dried tomato crostini

191

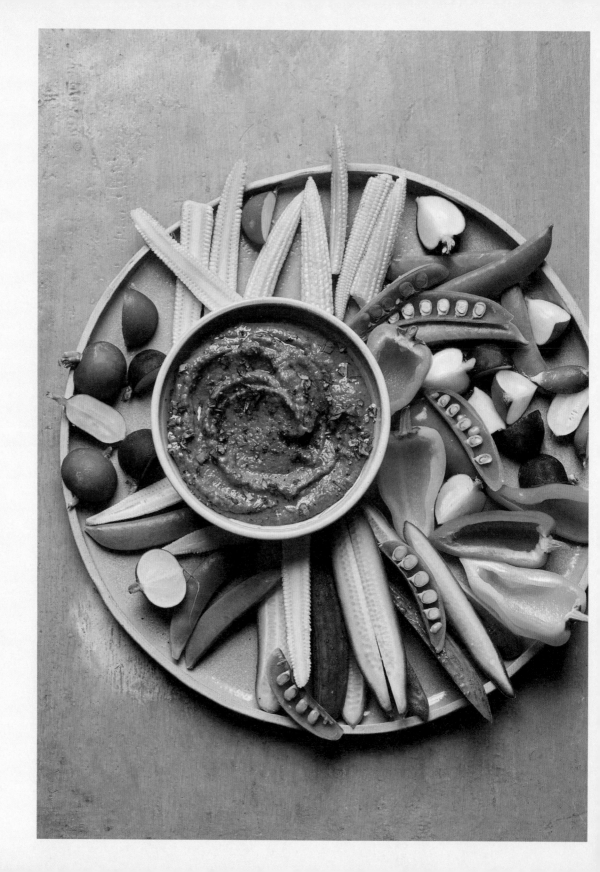

Red lentil *and* roasted red pepper dip

Serves 4
Prep 5 mins
Cook 30 mins

1 red pepper, seeded
  and halved
1 garlic clove, thinly sliced
2 tbsp extra-virgin olive oil,
  divided
$^1/_3$ cup (60g) dried red
  lentils
8fl oz (230ml) low-sodium
  vegetable stock
1 bay leaf
1 tsp tomato paste
1 tsp smoked paprika
6 walnuts
1 tsp lemon juice
handful of cilantro leaves,
  chopped
crudités, to serve—1 whole
  wheat tortilla, cut into
  triangles and baked; 1
  pepper, seeded and cut
  into strips; ½ cucumber,
  cut into strips; chopped
  radishes; snap peas;
  baby corn

**supports ovulatory health • aids egg and
sperm health • provides antioxidants**

Lentils supply plant-based protein, thought to
be beneficial for healthy ovulation. Sweet red
peppers add vitamin C; crunchy walnuts supply
omega-3s; while the colorful crudités add a range
of antioxidants.

Preheat the oven to 400°F (180°C). Place the red
pepper and garlic on a baking sheet and drizzle over
1 tablespoon of the olive oil. Roast for 20–30 minutes,
until softened.

In the meantime, place the lentils, stock, and bay leaf
in a saucepan. Bring to a boil, reduce to a simmer,
and cook for 25 minutes. Allow the pepper and lentils
to cool for 15 minutes. Remove the bay leaf.

Place the red pepper, garlic, lentils, the remaining
tablespoon of olive oil, the tomato paste, paprika,
walnuts, and lemon juice in a food processor and
pulse for about 1 minute, until a smooth consistency.

Place the lentil mixture in a bowl, sprinkle the cilantro
leaves over, then enjoy with crudités of choice. Leftover
dip can be stored in an airtight container in the fridge
for up to 3 days.

Sweet bites
and desserts

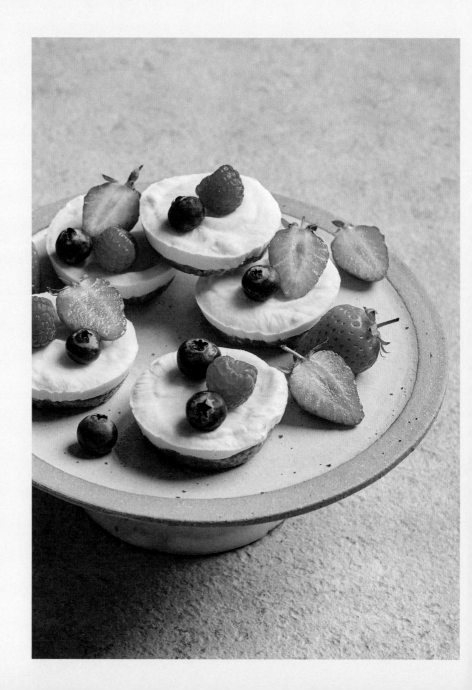

A fertility-friendly diet aims to reduce overall sugar to avoid rises in blood sugar levels that, over time, can potentially disrupt your hormones. However, a homemade sweet bite or dessert with nutritious ingredients can be a pleasurable part of your fertility diet—completing a weekend meal or get-together with friends and family, or simply enjoyed as an occasional treat.

The following selection of delicious sweet bites and desserts swaps processed sugars with naturally sweet fruit and mild spices and adds creamy, crumbly, and chewy textures with velvety yogurt, crunchy nuts, and soft oats. Different diets are considered, with flex options showing you how to convert dairy-based recipes into vegan-friendly ones.

Choose from mouthwatering fruit-based desserts, tangy and tasty frozen yogurt, and irresistible mini cheesecakes. Or enjoy a tasty banana bite or fruit and nut mix.

Spiced stoned fruit

aids egg and sperm health • may support implantation

This lightly spiced, naturally sweet dessert provides fiber, iron, and vitamins A, C, and E, promoting egg and sperm health. Brazil nuts add selenium, a key antioxidant that is also thought to support egg quality and healthy sperm parameters.

Serves 4
Prep 5 mins
Cook 20 mins

4 plums, halved and pitted
4 apricots, halved and pitted
1 tsp vanilla extract
juice of 1 lime
1 tsp pumpkin pie spice

To serve
18oz (500g) Greek yogurt
2 tbsp ground flaxseed
8 Brazil nuts, crushed

Heat the oven to 425°F (200°C). Add the fruit to a baking dish, along with the vanilla extract, lime, and pumpkin pie spice. Stir to combine.

Roast the fruit for 20 minutes, until the fruit has softened and the juices have formed a sticky sauce. Serve with Greek yogurt, topped with the flaxseeds and Brazil nuts. Any leftover cooked fruit can be stored in the fridge for up to 5 days.

Flex it—*Use a plant-based alternative to Greek yogurt for a vegan dessert.*

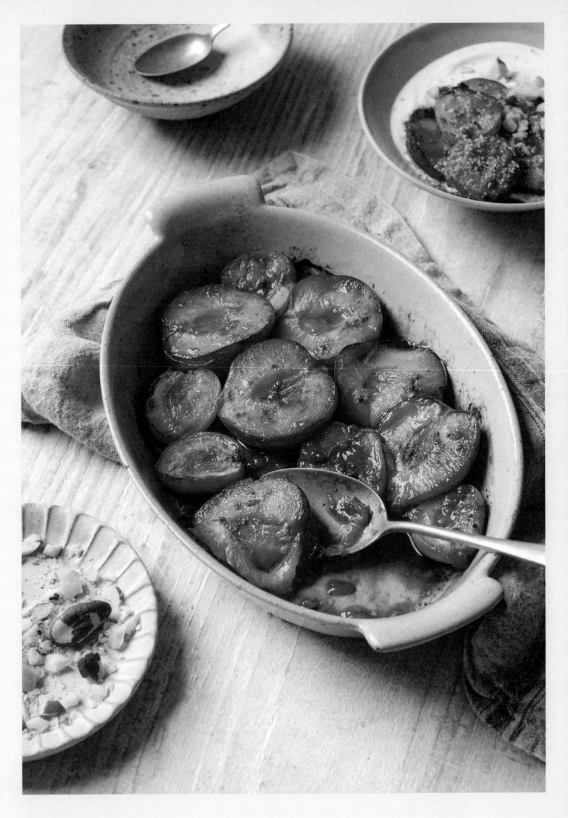

Spiced stoned fruit

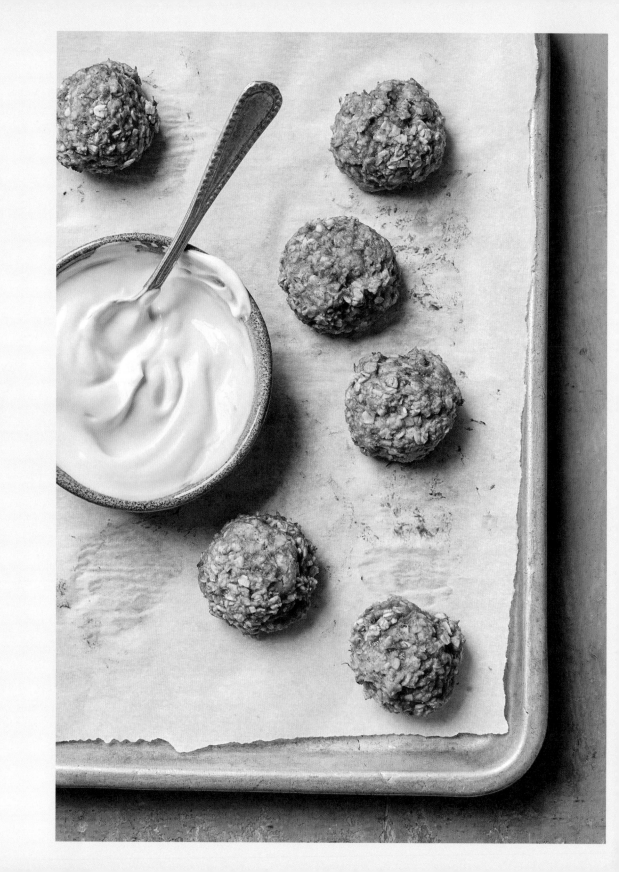

Banana bites

Makes 6
Prep 5 mins
Cook 15 mins
Cool 10 mins

1 large banana
1 tbsp unsalted crunchy
   peanut butter
$\frac{1}{2}$ cup (50g) rolled oats
$\frac{1}{2}$ tsp ground cinnamon
$\frac{1}{2}$ tsp vanilla extract
$\frac{1}{3}$ cup Greek yogurt,
   to serve

Flex it—*Use a plant-based
alternative to Greek yogurt for
a vegan bite.*

**supplies fibre • promotes hormonal balance
• provides antioxidants**

These flavorful bites are a nutritious treat. Fiber from the bananas and oats help to steady blood sugar levels, and healthy fats are supplied by peanut butter, all of which help steady hormones. Bananas also supply vitamins B6 and C, which may support progesterone levels.

Preheat the oven to 400°F (180°C) and line a baking sheet with parchment paper. Mash the banana in a large bowl. Stir in the peanut butter, oats, cinnamon, and vanilla extract and mix together with a spoon.

Using a tablespoon, spoon 6 scoops of the mixture onto the lined baking sheet, leaving a little room around each scoop. Place in the oven and bake for 15 minutes.

Allow the bites to cool for at least 10 minutes, then enjoy warm or cold, with a spoonful of yogurt. Any leftover bites can be stored in an airtight container for up to 3 days.

Full-of-fruit frozen yogurt

Serves 4
Prep 5 mins

11oz (320g) frozen berries
  of choice
1 sliced banana, frozen
14oz (400g) Greek yogurt
$\frac{1}{2}$ tsp vanilla extract
handful of almonds, chopped

provides antioxidants • aids egg and sperm health • nourishes the uterus

Tangy, sweet, and delicious, this palate-cleansing yogurt is packed with antioxidants, supporting progesterone levels and egg and sperm health. Almonds add crunch and extra vitamin E, important for uterine health.

Place all the ingredients except the almonds in a blender and blend on high for up to 1 minute, until well combined and a smooth consistency.

Spoon into 4 bowls, sprinkle the almonds on top, and enjoy right away.

200

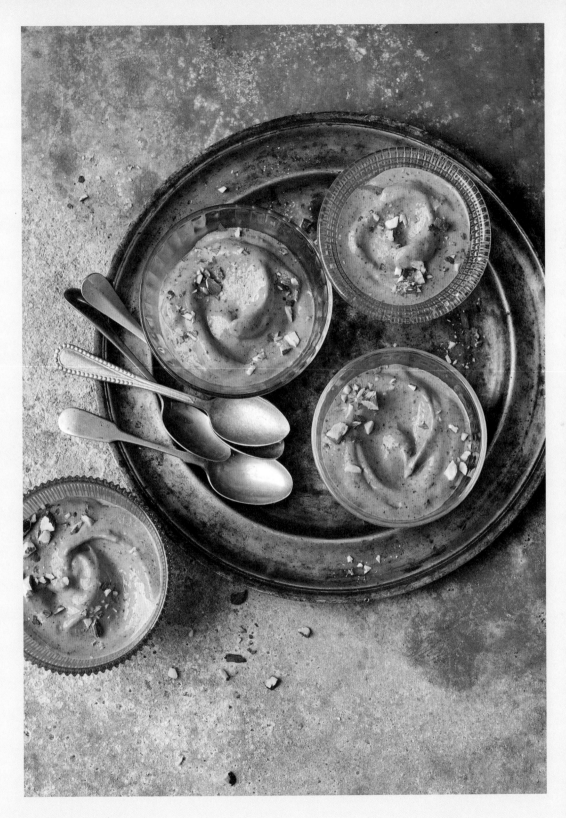

Full-of-fruit frozen yogurt

Fruit *and* nut mix

Makes 4 helpings
Prep 5 mins
Cook 10 mins

¼ cup (30g) pecans
¼ cup (30g) cashews
¼ cup (30g) almonds
½ tsp ground cinnamon
1 tbsp pumpkin seeds
1 tbsp sunflower seeds
1½ tbsp (10g) dried goji
   berries, chopped
1 tbsp (10g) dried apricots,
   chopped
handful of plain, unsalted
   popcorn

provides antioxidants • has anti-inflammatory properties • supplies fiber • aids egg and sperm health

Dried fruits add a juicy sweetness to this mix. Goji berries and apricots are full of fertility-promoting nutrients, including lycopene, iron, vitamins A, C, and E, and fiber. A selection of nuts adds plant-based protein, healthy fats, zinc, and extra vitamin E.

Preheat the oven to 375°F (170°C). Arrange the pecans, cashews, and almonds on a baking sheet, sprinkle with cinnamon, and toast in the oven for 10 minutes, until they release their aromas.

Once cool, place the nuts in an airtight container along with the pumpkin seeds, sunflower seeds, goji berries, apricots, and popcorn and mix together to combine. Store for up to 1 month.

Stewed apple *with* almond topping

Serves 2
Prep 5 mins
Cook 10 mins

1 tbsp olive oil
¹⁄₃ cup (30g) rolled oats
½ tsp ground cinnamon
¼ cup (30g) almonds, crushed
½ tsp vanilla extract
1 tbsp almond butter
1 tsp sunflower seeds
2 apples, peeled, cored, and diced
½ tsp ground nutmeg
2 tbsp pumpkin seeds, to garnish
9oz (250g) Greek yogurt, to serve

supplies fiber • supports healthy ovulation • supports male hormones

This gently spiced, sweet and nutty dessert is a flavorsome treat. Apples and oats deliver fiber, aiding gut health and ovulation; almonds supply vitamin E; and pumpkin seeds add zinc, promoting ovulation and, in men, healthy hormone levels.

Place the olive oil, oats, cinnamon, almonds, vanilla extract, almond butter, and sunflower seeds in a saucepan and heat gently for 5–10 minutes, until the oats have softened.s

In the meantime, place the apple and nutmeg in a small lidded saucepan with a splash of water. Cover and cook over a low-medium heat for about 10 minutes, until the apples have softened.

Spoon the stewed apple into 2 bowls and sprinkle over the almond topping. Sprinkle with the pumpkin seeds and serve with a spoonful of yogurt on the side.

(photographed overleaf)

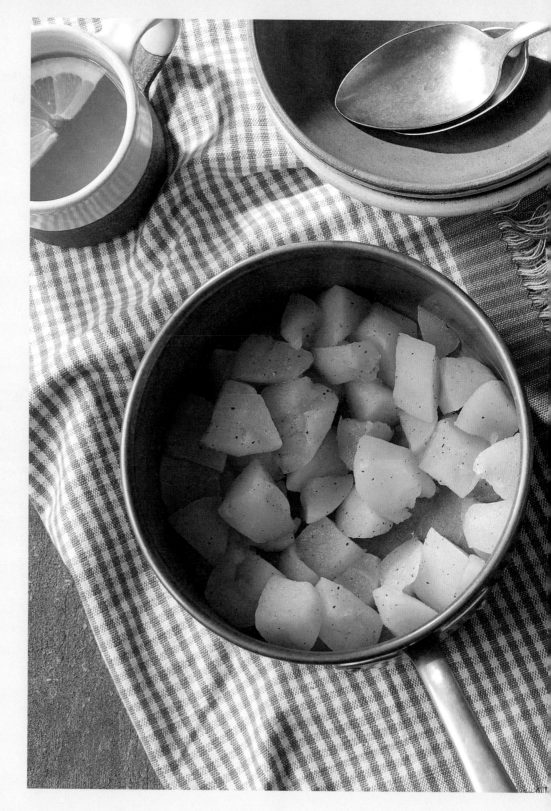

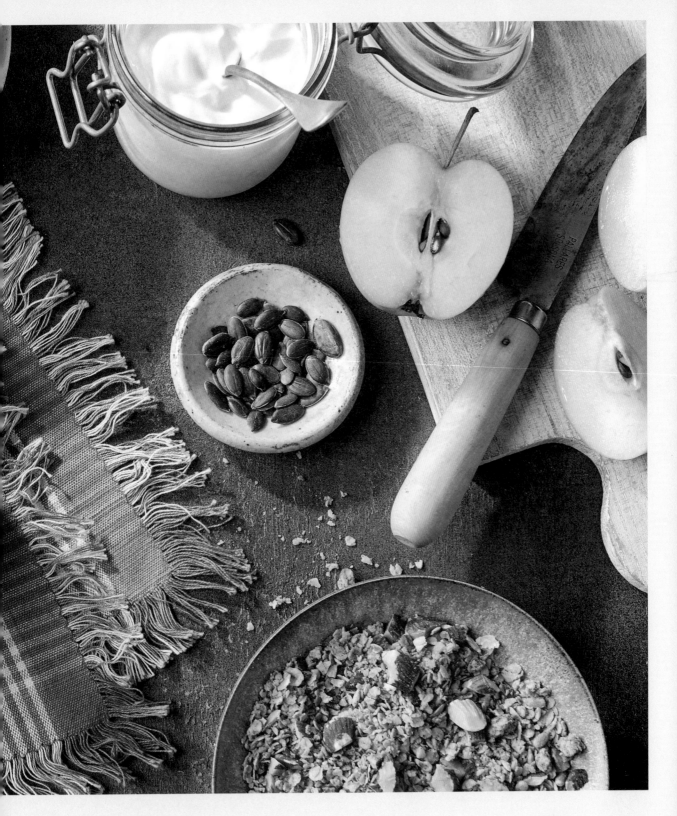

Stewed apple with almond topping

Mini berry cheesecakes

Makes 10
Prep 10 mins
Cook 15 mins

1 cup (160g) dried dates
³/₄ cup (100g) walnuts
9oz (250g) Greek yogurt
2 tbsp full-fat cream cheese
1 tbsp lemon juice
1 tsp vanilla extract
handful of fresh berries
** of choice**

Flex it—*For vegan cheesecake, use a vegan yogurt and cream cheese substitute.*

promotes hormonal balance • provides antioxidants • aids egg and sperm health

A creamy–crunchy combo, these hard to resist bites deliver plenty of fiber for a low GI treat to steady blood sugars, insulin, and other hormones. Walnuts have omega-3s, while berries add antioxidants, both supporting egg and sperm health.

Lightly grease a muffin pan and, if you wish, line with parchment paper to make it easier to remove the cheesecake cups. Place the dates and walnuts in a food processor and pulse until the mixture can be squeezed into a ball with your hands. Scoop out the mixture and push into the muffin pan cups, pressing evenly to form a base. Transfer to the freezer for about 1 hour, until firm.

Place the yogurt, cream cheese, lemon juice, and vanilla extract in a bowl and stir until creamy and smooth. Add 1 tablespoon of this creamy mixture to the top of each date and walnut base and spread it out evenly.

Return to the freezer for another 15 minutes, then remove the cheesecake cups, top with the berries, and serve. If preferred, take the pan out of the freezer 5 minutes before serving to allow the cups to soften first.

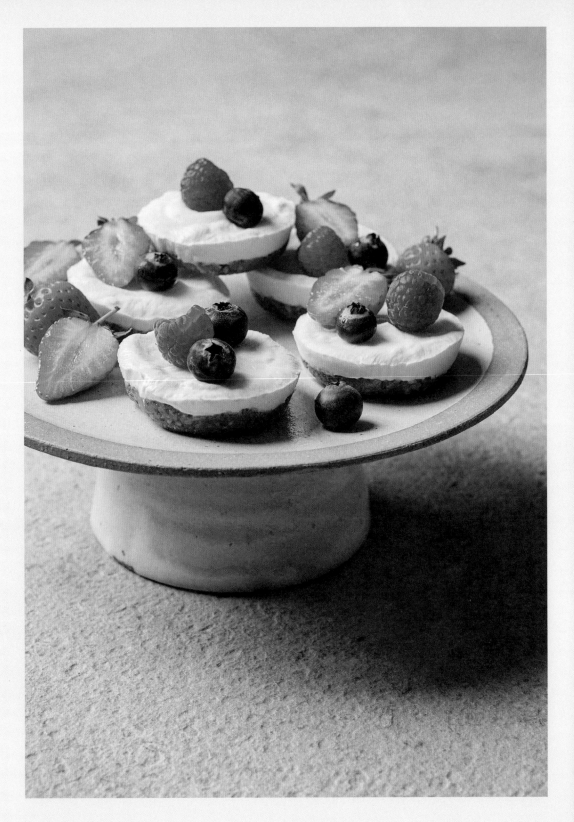

Mini berry cheesecakes

Drinks

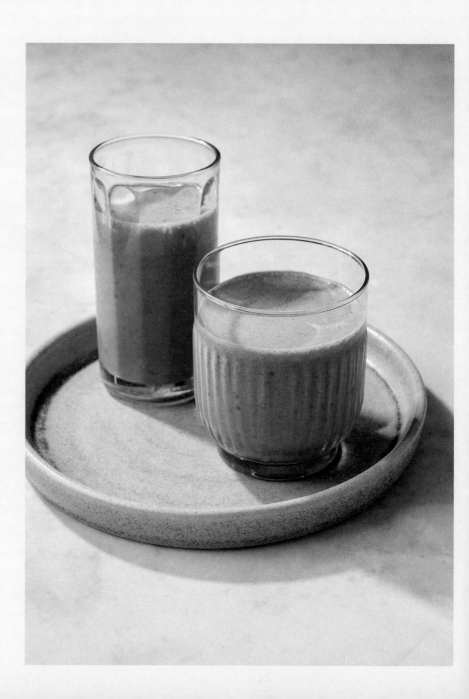

Staying well hydrated is fundamental to overall health and well-being and helps support fertility. Keeping your fluid intake up by drinking water throughout the day is the healthiest way to ensure that your body is adequately hydrated. If you prefer a little extra flavor, add a slice of lemon, lime, or cucumber.

For a warm beverage or more variety, the following recipes offer flavorful caffeine-free alternatives to water. Try replacing your morning coffee with warming aromatic spiced milk. Or enjoy nourishing drinks, such as apricot lassi, blackberry and ginger kefir, or peanut butter milkshake. These delicious nutritious beverages will perfectly complement your fertility diet.

Golden-spiced milk

provides key antioxidants • has anti-inflammatory properties • may support ovulatory health

This aromatic, slightly nutty, spiced milk makes a delicious caffeine-free warming beverage. Almond butter supplies some vitamin E; ginger adds anti-inflammatory and antioxidant properties; and whole milk may support ovulation.

Makes 1
Prep 5 mins
Cook 5–10 mins

9fl oz (250ml) milk or plant-based alternative
1 tsp almond butter
½ tsp vanilla extract

½ tsp ground cinnamon
¼ tsp ground turmeric
1in (2.5cm) piece of ginger, peeled and chopped
2 cardamom pods, lightly crushed
3 whole peppercorns

Place all the ingredients in a small saucepan over low heat. Gently simmer for 5–10 minutes.

Strain through a sieve before pouring into a cup. Enjoy warm.

Apricot lassi

**provides antioxidants • aids egg and sperm health
• nourishes the uterus • may support ovulatory health**

Sweet and gently spiced, this classic Indian drink is rich in antioxidants. Brightly colored apricots supply beta-carotene and vitamins A and E, supporting egg, sperm, uterine, and embryo health. Whole milk and yogurt may support ovulation and also provide fertility-supporting iodine and vitamin B12.

Makes 1
Prep 5 mins

¼ cup (30g) cashews (optional)
⅔ cup (125g) **Greek yogurt**
2 ripe apricots, pitted

3½fl oz (100ml) **milk or
  plant-based alternative**
pinch of ground ginger
pinch of ground cinnamon
ice, to serve (optional)

If using cashews, soak these in just-boiled water for at least 20 minutes, then drain.

Place the yogurt, apricots, milk, ginger, cinnamon, and cashews (if desired), in a blender. Blend until smooth. Pour into a glass, add ice if desired, and enjoy immediately.

Blackberry *and* ginger kefir

provides antioxidants • aids sperm health • may support progesterone levels

Slightly tangy with a sweet ginger kick, this refreshing drink is rich in vitamin C from the blackberries, supporting progesterone levels and thought to promote healthy sperm motility and shape and protect against sperm DNA damage. Kefir acts as a probiotic, supporting gut health.

Serves 2
Prep 5 mins

5¾oz (160g) blackberries
   (fresh or frozen)
1in (2.5cm) piece of ginger,
   peeled and diced
16fl oz (500ml) plain kefir
½ tsp vanilla extract
ice, to serve (optional)

Add all of the ingredients to a blender and blend to a smooth consistency. Pour into 2 glasses, add ice if desired, and enjoy!

Peanut butter milkshake

supports healthy ovulation • supplies fiber

Sweet and nutty, this delicious shake is packed with nutrients. Peanuts supply healthy polyunsaturated fats, as well as plant-based protein and fiber, both of which support ovulation. Bananas and oats top up the fiber content and add vital vitamins, selenium, zinc, and iron.

Serves 2
Prep 5 mins

1 banana
1 tbsp unsalted peanut butter
½ tsp vanilla extract
14fl oz (400ml) milk or
    plant-based alternative
2 tbsp Greek yogurt
1 tbsp rolled oats

Place all of the ingredients in a blender and blend to a smooth consistency. Pour into 2 glasses and enjoy right away!

Index

Bibliography

10–11 Menstrual cycle

Cable JK, Girder MH, "Physiology, progesterone," *StatPearls*, 2022.

Diedrich et al, "The role of the endometrium and embryo in human implantation," *Hum Reprod Update*, 2007; 13(4): 365–377. doi: 10.1093/humupd/dmm011

Draper CF et al, "Menstrual cycle rhythmicity: metabolic patterns in healthy women," *Sci Rep*, 2018; 8(14568). doi: 10.1038/s41598-018-32647-0

NHS, "Periods and fertility in the menstrual cycle" (online), 2019. www.nhs/conditions/periods/fertility-in-the-menstrual-cycle/

Reed, BG, Carr, BR, "The normal menstrual cycle and control of ovulation," *Nat Lib Med*, 2018. www.ncbi.nlm.nih.gov/books/NBK279054/

12–13 Monitoring menstrual cycle

NHS, "Ovulation pain" (online), 2019. www.nhs.uk/conditions/ovulation-pain/

Roney JR, Simmons ZL, "Hormonal predictors of sexual motivation in natural menstrual cycles" *Horm Behav*, 2013; 63(4): 636–45. doi: 0.1016/j.yhbeh.2013.02.013

Steward K, Raja A, "Physiology, ovulation, and basal body temperature," *StatPearls*, 2022. PMID: 31536292

14–15 Men's reproduction/sperm

O'Donnell L, Stanton P, de Krester DM, "Endocrinology of the male reproductive system and spermatogenesis," MDText.com, Inc. Last updated 2017

WHO, "Examination and processing of human semen" (online), 2021. www.who.int/publications/i/item/9789240030787

16–17 Fertility problems

Agarwal A et al, "A unique view on male infertility around the globe," *Reprod Biol Endocrinol*, 2015; 13(37). doi: 10.1186/s12958-015-0032-1

BMJ Best Practice, "Male factor infertility" (online), 2022. www.bestpractice.bmj.com/topics/en-gb/497#referencePop1

Leaver RB, "Male infertility: an overview of causes and treatment options," *Br J Nurs*, 2016; 13; 25(18): S35 –S40. doi: 10.12968/bjon.2016.25.18.S35

WHO, "Infertility" (online), 2020. www.who.int/news-room/fact-sheets/detail/infertility

18 PCOS

NHS, "Polycystic ovary syndrome" (online), 2019. www.nhs.uk/conditions/polycystic-ovary-syndrome-pcos/

Rotterdam ESHRE/ASRM-Sponsored PCOS Consensus Workshop Group,

"Revised 2003 consensus on diagnostic criteria and long-term health risks related to polycystic ovary syndrome," *Fertil Steril*, 2004 Jan; 81(1): 19–25. doi: 10.1016/j.fertnstert.2003.10.004

19 Thyroid problems

British Thyroid Foundation, "Pregnancy and fertility in thyroid disorders" (online), 2021. www.btf-thyroid.org/pregnancy-and-fertility-in-thyroid-disorders

Mintziori G et al, "Consequences of hyperthyroidism in male and female fertility: pathophysiology and current management," *J Endcrinol Invest*, 2016; 39 (8): 849–53. doi: 10.1007/s40618-016-0452-6

Verma I et al, "Prevalence of hypothyroidism in infertile women and evaluation of response of treatment for hypothyroidism on infertility," *IntJ Appl Basic Med Res*, 2012; Jan 2(1): 17–19. doi: 10.4103/2229-516X.96795

19 Diabetes

Guo-Lian D et al, "The effects of diabetes on male fertility and epigenetic regulation during spermatogenesis," *Asian J Androl*, 2015 Nov–Dec; 17(6): 948–53. doi: 10.4103/1008-682X.150844

Thong EP et al, "Diabetes: a metabolic and reproductive disorder in women," *The Lancet*, 2019; 8(2): 134–149. DOI: 10.1016/S2213-8587(19)30345-6

Your fertility, "Diabetes" (online), 2022. www.yourfertility.org.au/everyone/health-medical/diabetes

20 Celiac disease

Freeman HJ, "Reproductive changes associated with celiac disease," *World J Gastroenterol*, 2010 Dec 14; 16(46): 5810–14. doi: 10.3748/wjg.v16.i46.5810

Tersigni C et al, "Celiac disease and reproductive disorders: meta-analysis of epidemiologic associations and potential pathogenic mechanisms," *Hum Reprod Update*, 2014; 20(4): 582–93. doi: 10.1093/humupd/dmu007

22–23 Age and fertility

Appiah D et al, "Trends in age at natural menopause and reproductive life span among US women, 1959–2018," *Am Med Assoc*, 2021; 325(13): 1328-30. doi:10.1001/jama.2021.0278

Delbaere I et al, "Knowledge about the impact of age on fertility," *Ups J Med Sci*, 2020; 125(2): 167–74. doi: 10.1080/03009734.2019.1707913

Wallace WHB, Kelsey TW, "Human ovarian reserve from conception to the menopause," *PLoS One*, 2010. doi: 10.1371/journal.pone.0008772

24 BMI and diet

Bain H et al, "Male waist circumference in relation to semen quality and partner infertility treatment outcomes among couples undergoing infertility treatment with assisted reproductive technologies," *Am J Clin Nutr*, 2022; 115 (3): 833–842. doi: 10.1093/ajcn/nqab364

Metwally, M et al, "Does high body mass index increase the risk of miscarriage after spontaneous and assisted conception?," *Fertil Steril*, 2008; 90(3): 714–26. doi: 10.1016/j.fertnstert.2007.07.1290

NICE, "Fertility problems: assessment and treatment" (online), 2017. www.nice.org.uk/guidance/cg156

Salas-Huetos A et al, "Male adiposity, sperm parameters and reproductive hormones," *Obes Rev*, 2021; 22(1): e13082. doi: 10.1111/obr.13082

Sasaki H et al, "Impact of oxidative stress on age-associated decline in oocyte developmental competence," *Front Endocrinol*, 2019; 10: 811. doi: 10.3389/fendo.2019.00811

Weiss G et al, "Inflammation in reproductive disorders," *Reprod Sci*, 2009; 16(2): 216–229. doi: 10.1177/1933719108330087

28–29 Poor diet, caffeine, alcohol

Hatch EE et al, "Intake of sugar-sweetened beverages and fecundability in a North American preconception cohort," *Epidemiology*, 2018; 29(3): 369–378. doi: 10.1097/EDE.0000000000000812

Kearns M et al, "The impact of non-caloric sweeteners on male fertility," *Proceedings of the Nutrition Society*, 2021; 80(OCE5): e167. doi: 10.1017/S0029665121002950

Laskowski D et al, "Insulin during in vitro oocyte maturation has an impact on development, mitochondria, and cytoskeleton in bovine day 8 blastocysts," *Theriogenology*, 2017; 101: 15–25. doi: 10.1016/j.theriogenology.2017.06.002

NHS, "Foods to avoid in pregnancy" (online), 2020. www.nhs.uk/pregnancy/keeping-well/foods-to-avoid/

Panth N et al, "The influence of diet on fertility and the implications for public health nutrition in the United States," *Front Public Health*, 2018; 6(211). doi: 10.3389/fpubh.2018.00211

Setti A et al, "Is there an association between artificial sweetener consumption and assisted reproduction outcomes?," *RBM Online*, 2018; 36(2):

145–53. doi: 10.1016/j.rbmo.2017.11.004
Fan D et al, "Female alcohol consumption and fecundability: a systematic review and dose-response meta-analysis," *Sc Rep*, 2017, 7, 13815. doi: 10.1038/s41598-017-14261-8
Ricci E et al, "Semen quality and alcohol intake," *Reprod Biomed Online*, 2017 Jan; 34(1): 38–47. doi: 10.1016/j.rbmo.2016.09.012
Sundermann AC et al, "Week-by-week alcohol consumption in early pregnancy and spontaneous abortion risk," *Am J Obstet Gynecol*, 2020; 224(1): 97.E1–97.E16. doi: 10.1016/j.ajog.2020.07.012
Sundermann AC et al, "Alcohol use in pregnancy and miscarriage," *Alcohol Clin Exp Res*, 2019; 43(8): 1606–16. doi: 10.1111/acer.14124
Van Heertum K, Rossi B, "Alcohol and fertility: how much is too much?," *Fertil Res Pract*, 2017; 3(10). doi: 10.1186/s40738-017-0037-x
Greenwood DC et al, "Caffeine intake during pregnancy and adverse birth outcomes," *Eur J Epidemiol*, 2014; 29(10): 725–34. doi: 10.1007/s10654-014-9944-x
James JE, "Maternal caffeine consumption and pregnancy outcomes: a narrative review with implications for advice to mothers and mothers-to-be," *BMJ* 2021; 26: 114–15.
NHS, "Breastfeeding and diet" (online, caffeine amounts), 2018. www.nhs.uk/conditions/baby/breastfeeding-and-bottle-feeding/breastfeeding-and-lifestyle/diet/
Ricci E et al, "Coffee and caffeine intake and male infertility," *Nutr J*, 2017; 24; 16(1): 37. doi: 10.1186/s12937-017-0257-2

30–31 Smoking, meds, EDCs
de Angelis C et al, "Smoke, alcohol and drug addiction and female fertility," *Reprod Biol Endocrinol*, 2020; 18: 21. doi: 10.1186/s12958-020-0567-7
Dorfman SF, "Tobacco and fertility: our responsibilities," *Fertil Steril*, 2008; 89(3): 502–4. doi: 10.1016/j.fertnstert.2008.01.011
Firns S et al, "The effect of cigarette smoking, alcohol consumption and fruit and vegetable consumption on IVF outcomes," *Reprod Biol Endocrinol*, 2015; 6(13): 134. doi: 10.1186/s12958-015-0133-x
Künzle R et al, "Semen quality of male smokers and nonsmokers in infertile couples," *Fertil Steril*, 2003; 79(2): 287–91. doi: 10.1016/s0015-0282(02)04664-2
Sansone A et al, "Smoke, alcohol and drug addiction and male fertility," *Reprod Biol Endocrinol*, 2018; 16:3. doi: 10.1186/s12958-018-0320-7
Szumilas K et al, "The effects of

e-cigarette vapor components on the morphology and function of the male and female reproductive systems," *Int J Environ Res Pub Health*, 2020; 17(17): 6152. doi: 10.3390/ijerph17176152
Whitaker DL et al, "Anabolic steroid misuse and male infertility: management and strategies to improve patient awareness," *Expert Rev Endocrinol Metab*, 2021; 16(3). doi: 10.1080/17446651.2021.1921574
Hartle JC et al, "The consumption of canned food and beverages and urinary Bisphenol A concentrations in NHANES 2003–2008," *Environ Res*, 2016; 150: 375–82. doi: 10.1016/j.envres.2016.06.008
Ingaramo P et al, "Are glyphosate and glyphosate-based herbicides endocrine disruptors that alter female fertility?," *Mol Cell Endocrinol*, 2020; 1(518): 110934. doi: 10.1016/j.mce.2020.110934
Krzastek SC et al, "Impact of environmental toxin exposure on male fertility potential," *Transl Androl Urol*, 2020; 9(6): 2797–813. doi: 10.21037/tau-20-685
López-Botella A et al, "Impact of heavy metals on human male fertility," *Antioxidants*, 2021 Sep 15; 10(9): 1473. doi: 10.3390/antiox10091473
Pivonello C et al, "Bisphenol A: an emerging threat to female fertility," *Reprod Biol Endocrinol*, 2020; 14; 18(1): 22. doi: 10.1186/s12958-019-0558-8
Vessa B et al, "Endocrine disruptors and female fertility: a review of pesticide and plasticizer effects," *F&S Reports*, 2022; 3(2): 86–90. doi: 10.1016/j.xfre.2022.04.003
WHO, "Identification of risks from exposure to endocrine-disrupting chemicals" (online), 2014. www.who.int/europe/publications/i/item/9789289050142

34–35 Diet: eggs and ovarian reserve
KaboodMehri R et al, "The association between the levels of anti-Müllerian hormone (AMH) and dietary intake in Iranian women," *Arch Gynecol Obstet*, 2021; 304(3): 687–94. doi: 10.1007/s00404-021-06098-4
Kadir, M et al, "Folate intake and ovarian reserve among women attending a fertility center," *Fertil Steril*, 2022; 117(1): 171–80. doi: 10.1016/j.fertnstert.2021.09.037
Mínguez-Alarcón, L et al, "Hair mercury levels, intake of omega-3 fatty acids and ovarian reserve among women attending a fertility center," *Inter J Hyg Environ Health*, 2021; 237 (113825). doi:10.1016/j.ijheh.2021.113825
Moslehi N et al, "Do dietary intakes influence the rate of decline in anti-Müllerian hormone among eumenorrheic women?," *Nutr J*, 2019;

18(83). doi: 10.1186/s12937-019-0508-5
Moy V et al, "Obesity adversely affects serum anti-müllerian hormone (AMH) levels in Caucasian women," *J Assist Reprod Genet*, 2015; 32(9): 1305–11. doi: 10.1007/s10815-015-0538-7
Safiyeh FD et al, "The effect of selenium and vitamin E supplementation on anti-Müllerian hormone and antral follicle count in infertile women with occult premature ovarian insufficiency," *Complement Ther Med*, 2021; 56 (102533). doi: 10.1016/j.ctim.2020.102533

35 Diet: sperm health
Amann RP, "The Cycle of the Seminiferous Epithelium in Humans: A Need to Revisit?," *J Androl*, 2013; 189. doi: 10.2164/jandrol.107.004655
Natt D et al, "Human sperm displays rapid responses to diet," *PLoS*, 2019. doi: 10.1371/journal.pbio.3000559

36–37 Diet: implantation, conception, and pregnancy
Chiu YH et al, "Serum omega-3 fatty acids and treatment outcomes among women undergoing assisted reproduction," *Hum Reprod*, 2018; 33(10): 156–65. doi: 10.1093/humrep/dex335
Cicek N et al, "Vitamin E effect on controlled ovarian stimulation of unexplained infertile women," *J Assist Reprod Genet*, 2012; 29(4). doi: 10.1007/s10815-012-9747-5
Gaskins AJ et al, "Maternal wholegrain intake and outcomes of IVF," *Fertil Steril*, 2017; 105(6): 1503–1510.E4. doi: 10.1016/j.fertnstert.2016.02.015
Gaskins AJ et al, "The impact of dietary folate intake on reproductive function in premenopausal women," *PloS One*, 2012; 7(9): e46276. doi: 10.1371/journal.pone.0046276
Halpern G et al, "Beetroot, watermelon and ginger juice supplementation may increase the clinical outcomes of ICSI," *Fertil Steril*, 2019; 112(3). doi: 10.1016/j.fertnstert.2019.07.1334
Moreno I et al, "Evidence that the endometrial microbiota has an effect on implantation success or failure," *Am J Obstet Gynecol*, 2016; 215(6): 684–703. doi: 10.1016/j.ajog.2016.09.075
Mumford SL et al, "Serum antioxidants are associated with serum reproductive hormones and ovulation among healthy women," *J Nutr*, 2016; 146(1): 98–106. doi: 10.3945/jn.115.217620
Qazi IH et al, "Selenium, selenoproteins, and female reproduction," *Molecules*, 2018; 22; 23(12): 3053. doi: 10.3390/molecules23123053

Bala R, "Hyperhomocysteinemia and low vitamin B12 are associated with the risk of early pregnancy loss," *Nutr Res*, 2021; 91: 57–66. doi: 10.1016/j.nutres.2021.05.002

Duntas LH, "Selenium and at-risk pregnancy: challenges and controversies," *Thyroid Res*, 2020; 13(16). doi: 10.1186/s13044-020-00090-x

Gaskins AJ et al, "Maternal prepregnancy folate intake and risk of spontaneous abortion and stillbirth," *Obstet Gynecol*, 2014; 124(1): 22–31. doi: 10.1097/AOG.0000000000000343

Radzinsky VE et al, "Vitamin D insufficiency as a risk factor for reproductive losses in miscarriage," *Gyne Endocrinol*, 2021; 37(1): 8–12. doi: 10.1080/09513590.2021.2006451

38–41 The Mediterranean diet

Gaskins AJ et al, "Maternal whole grain intake and outcomes of IVF," *Fertil Steril*, 2016; 105(6): 1503–10.e4. doi: 10.1016/j.fertnstert.2016.02.015

Karayiannis D et al, "Adherence to the Mediterranean diet and IVF success rate among non-obese women attempting fertility," *Hum Reprod*, 2018; 1; 33(3): 494–502. doi: 10.1093/humrep/dey003

Kermack A et al, "Effect of a 6-week 'Mediterranean' dietary intervention on in vitro human embryo development," *Fertil Steril*, 2020; 113(2): 260–69. doi: 10.1016/j.fertnstert.2019.09.041

Mumford SL et al, "Higher urinary lignan concentrations in women but not men are positively associated with shorter time to pregnancy," *J Nutr*, 2014; 144(3): 352–58. doi: 10.3945/jn.113.184820

Parisi F et al, "Periconceptional maternal 'high fish and olive oil, low meat' dietary pattern is associated with increased embryonic growth," *Ultrasound Obstet Gynecol*, 2017; 50(6): 709–16. doi: 10.1002/uog.17408

Ricci E et al, "Mediterranean diet and the risk of poor semen quality," *Andrology*, 2019; 7(2):156–62. doi: 10.1111/andr.12587

Russell JB et al, "Does dietary protein and carbohydrate intake influence blastocyst development and pregnancy rates?," *Fertil Steril*, 2012; 98(3): S233–34. doi: 10.1016/j.fertnstert.2012.07.849

Salas-Huetos A et al, "Effect of nut consumption on semen quality and functionality in healthy men consuming a Western-style diet," *Am J Clin Nutr*, 2018; 1;108(5): 953–62. doi: 10.1093/ajcn/nqy181

Skoracka K et al, "Female fertility and the nutritional approach: the most essential aspects," *Adv Nutr*, 2021; 12(6): 2372–386. doi: 10.1093/advances/nmab068

Sun H et al, "Mediterranean diet improves embryo yield in IVF," *Reprod Biol Endocrinol*, 2019; 17(73). doi: 10.1186/s12958-019-0520-9

Vujkovic M et al, "The preconception Mediterranean dietary pattern in couples undergoing in vitro fertilization/intracytoplasmic sperm injection treatment increases the chance of pregnancy," *Fertil Steril*, 2010; 94(6): 2096 –101. doi: 10.1016/j.fertnstert.2009.12.079

44 Protein

Afeiche MC et al, "Meat intake and reproductive parameters among young men," *Epidemiol*, 2014; 25(3): 323–30. doi: 10.1097/EDE.0000000000000092

Chavarro JE et al, "Protein intake and ovulatory infertility," *Am J Obstet Gynecol*, 2008; 198(2): 210.e1–7. doi: 10.1016/j.ajog.2007.06.057

Nassan FL et al, "Intake of protein-rich foods in relation to outcomes of infertility treatment with assisted reproductive technologies," *Am J Clin Nutr*, 2018; 108(5): 1104–12. doi: 10.1093/ajcn/nqy185

Russell JB et al, "Does dietary protein and carbohydrate intake influence blastocyst development and pregnancy rates?," *Fertil Steril*, 2012; 98(3): S233–34. doi: 10.1016/j.fertnstert.2012.07.849

Sorensen LB et al, "Effects of increased dietary protein-to-carbohydrate ratios in women with polycystic ovary syndrome," *Am J Clin Nutr*, 2012; 95(1): 39–48. doi: 10.3945/ajcn.111.020693

46 Soy and fertility

Chavarro JE et al, "Soy food and isoflavone intake in relation to semen quality parameters among men from an infertility clinic," *Hum Reprod*, 2008; 23(11): 2584–90. doi: 10.1093/humrep/den243

Jefferson WN, "Adult ovarian function can be affected by high levels of soy," *J Nutr*, 2010; 140(12): 2322S–2325S. doi: 10.3945/jn.110.123802Nassan

Reed KE et al, "Neither soy nor isoflavone intake affects male reproductive hormones," *Reprod Toxicol*, 2021; 100: 60–67. doi: 10.1016/j.reprotox.2020.12.019

Rizzo G et al, "The role of soy and soy isoflavones on women's fertility and related outcomes," *J Nutr Sci*, 2022; 11(17). doi: 10.1017/jns.2022.15

Vanegas JC et al, "Soy food intake and treatment outcomes of women undergoing assisted reproductive technology," *Fertil Steril*, 2015; 103(3): 749–55.e2. doi: 10.1016/j.fertnstert.2014.12.104

Wesselink AK et al, "Dietary phytoestrogen intakes of adult women are not strongly related to fecundability," *J Nutr*, 2020; 1;150(5): 1240–51. doi: 10.1093/jn/nxz335

47 Dairy and fertility

Afeiche MC et al, "Dairy intake and semen quality among men attending a fertility clinic," *Fertil Steril*, 2014; 101(5): 1280–87. doi: 10.1016/j.fertnstert.2014.02.003

Bordoni A et al, "Dairy products and inflammation," *Food Sc Nutr*, 2017; 57 (12). doi: 10.1080/10408398.2014.967385

Chavarro JE et al, "A prospective study of dairy foods intake and anovulatory infertility," *Hum Reprod*, 2007; 22(5): 1340–47. doi: 10.1093/humrep/dem019

49–50 Carbohydrates

Chavarro JE et al, "A prospective study of dietary carbohydrate quantity and quality in relation to risk of ovulatory infertility," *Eur J Clin Nutr*, 2009; 63(1): 78–86. doi: 10.1038/sj.ejcn.1602904

McGrice M, Porter J, "The effect of low carbohydrate diets on fertility hormones and outcomes in overweight and obese women," *Nutrients*, 2017; 9(3): 204. doi: 10.3390/nu9030204

Willis SK, "Glycemic load, dietary fiber, and added sugar and fecundability in 2 preconception cohorts," *Am J Clin Nutr*, 2020; 112(1): 27–38. doi: 10.1093/ajcn/nqz312

50 Gluten

Dhalwani NN et al, "Women with celiac disease present with fertility problems no more often than women in the general population," *Gastroenterology*, 2014; 147(6): 1267–74.e1; quiz e13–14. doi: 10.1053/j.gastro.2014.08.025

Marziali M et al, "Gluten-free diet: a new strategy for management of painful endometriosis related symptoms?," *Minerva Surgery*, 2012; 67(6): 499–504. PMID: 23334113

Pieczynska J, "Do celiac disease and non-celiac gluten sensitivity have the same effects on reproductive disorders?," *Nutrition*, 2018; 48: 18–23. doi: 10.1016/j.nut.2017.11.022

52–53 Blood sugar/GI levels

Saadati N et al, "The effect of low glycemic index diet on the reproductive and clinical profile in women with polycystic ovarian syndrome," *Heliyon*, 2021; 7(11): e08338. PMID: 34820542

University of Sydney, "Glycemic index research and GI news" (online), 2022. www.glycemicindex.com/gi-search/

Willis SK et al, "Glycemic load, dietary fiber, and added sugar and fecundability," *Am J Clin Nutr*, 2020; 1; 112(1): 27–38. doi: 10.1093/ajcn/nqz312

54–55 Fats

Chavarro JE, "Dietary fatty acid intakes and the risk of ovulatory infertility," *Am J Clin Nutr*, 2007; 85(1): 231–7. doi: 10.1093/ajcn/85.1.231

Jensen TA et al, "High dietary intake of saturated fat is associated with reduced semen quality among 701 young Danish men from the general population," *Am J Clin Nutr*, 2013; 97(2): 411–8. doi: 10.3945/ajcn.112.042432

Kim K et al, "Associations between preconception plasma fatty acids and pregnancy outcomes," *Epidemiol*, 2019; 30(2): S37–S46. doi: 10.1097/EDE.0000000000001066

Nehra D et al, "Prolonging the female reproductive lifespan and improving egg quality with dietary omega-3 fatty acids," *Aging Cell*, 2012; 11(6): 1046–54. doi: 10.1111/acel.12006

56–59 Fruits and vegetables

Alahmar AT, "Role of oxidative stress in male infertility," *J Hum Reprod Sci*, 2019; 21(1): 4–18. doi: 10.4103/jhrs.JHRS_150_18

Durairajanayagam D et al, "Lycopene and male infertility," *Asian J Androl*, 2014; 16(3): 420–25. doi: 10.4103/1008-682X.126384

Maconochie N et al, "Risk factors for first trimester miscarriage," *BJOG*, 2007; 114(2): 170–86. doi: 10.1111/j.1471-0528.2006.01193.x

NHS, "5 a day portion sizes" (online), 2022; www.nhs.uk/live-well/eat-well/5-a-day/5-a-day-what-counts/

Nouri M et al, "The effects of lycopene supplement on the spermatogram and seminal oxidative stress in infertile men," *Phytother Res*, 2019; 33(12): 3203–11. doi: 10.1002/ptr.6493

Ruder EH et al, "Female dietary antioxidant intake and time to pregnancy among couples treated for unexplained infertility," *Fertil Steril,* 2014; 101(3): 759–66. doi: 10.1016/j.fertnstert.2013.11.008

Showell MG et al, "Antioxidants for female subfertility," *Cochrane Database Syst Rev,* 2020; 8(8): CD007807. doi: 10.1002/14651858.CD007807.pub4

Wojsiat J et al, "The role of oxidative stress in female infertility and in vitro fertilization," *Postepy Hig Med Dosw*, 2017; 71(0): 359–66. doi: 10.5604/01.3001.0010.3820

60 Vitamin A

Clagett-Dame M, Knutson D, "Vitamin A in reproduction and development," *Nutrients*, 2011; 3(4): 385–428. doi: 10.3390/nu3040385

61–63 B vitamins

Abraham GE, "Nutritional factors in the etiology of the premenstrual tension syndromes," *J Reprod Med*, 1983; 28(7): 446–64. PMID: 6684167

Banihani SA, "Vitamin B12 and semen quality," *Biomolecules*, 2017; 9; 7(2): 42. doi: 10.3390/biom7020042

Bennett M, "Vitamin B12 deficiency, infertility and recurrent fetal loss," *J Reprod Med*, 2001; 46(3): 209–12. PMID: 11304860

Cirillo M et al, "5-methyltetrahydrofolate and vitamin B12 supplementation is associated with clinical pregnancy and live birth in women undergoing assisted reproductive technology," *Int J Environ Res Public Health*, 2021; 23; 18(23): 12280. doi: 10.3390/ijerph182312280

Gaskins AJ et al, "Maternal prepregnancy folate intake and risk of spontaneous abortion and stillbirth," *Obstet Gynecol*, 2014; 124(1): 23–31. doi: 10.1097/AOG.0000000000000343

Michels KA et al, "Folate, homocysteine and the ovarian cycle among healthy regularly menstruating women," *Hum Reprod*, 2017; 1;32(8): 1743–50. doi: 10.1093/humrep/dex233

Young SS et al, "The association of folate, zinc and antioxidant intake with sperm aneuploidy in healthy non-smoking men," *Hum Reprod*, 2008; 23(5): 1014–22. doi: 10.1093/humrep/den036

64–65 Vitamin C, D, E

Andersen LB et al, "Vitamin D insufficiency is associated with increased risk of first-trimester miscarriage in the Odense child cohort," *Am J Clin Nutr*, 2015; 102(3): 633–8. doi: 10.3945/ajcn.114.103655

Arab A et al, "The association between serum vitamin D, fertility and semen quality," *Int J Surg*, 2019; 71: 101–09. doi: 10.1016/j.ijsu.2019.09.025

Li M et al, "Men's intake of vitamin C and carotene is positively related to fertilization rate but not to live birth rate in couples undergoing infertility treatment," *Journ Nutr*, 2019; 149(11): 1977–1984. doi: 10.1093/jn/nxz149

Gagne A et al, "Absorption, transport, and bioavailability of vitamin E and its role in pregnant women," *J Obstet Gynaecol Can*, 2009; 31(3): 210–7. doi: 10.1016/s1701-2163(16)34118-4

Greco E et al, "Reduction of the incidence of sperm DNA fragmentation by oral antioxidant treatment," *J Androl*, 2005; 26(3): 349–53. doi: 10.2164/jandrol.04146

Hashemi Z et al, "The effects of vitamin E supplementation on endometrial thickness, and gene expression of vascular endothelial growth factor and inflammatory cytokines among women with implantation failure," *J Matern Fetal Neonatal Med*, 2019; 32(1): 95–102. doi: 10.1080/14767058.2017.1372413

Irani M, Merhi Z, "Role of vitamin D in ovarian physiology and its implication in reproduction," *Fertil Steril*, 2014; 102(2): 460–68.e3. doi: 10.1016/j.fertnstert.2014.04.046

Jukic AMZ et al, "Pre-conception 25-hydroxyvitamin D (25(OH)D) and fecundability," *Hum Reprod*, 2019; 34(11): 2163–72. doi: 10.1093/humrep/dez170

Mumford SL et al, "Serum antioxidants are associated with serum reproductive hormones and ovulation among healthy women," *J Nutr*, 2016; 146(1): 98–106. doi: 10.3945/jn.115.217620

Ruder EH et al, "Female dietary antioxidant intake and time to pregnancy among couples treated for unexplained infertility," *Fertil Steril*, 2014; 101(3): 759–66. doi: 10.1016/j.fertnstert.2013.11.008

66 Selenium

Ashan U et al, "Role of selenium in male reproduction," *Anim Reprod Sci*, 2014; 146(1–2) :55–62. doi: 10.1016/j.anireprosci.2014.01.009

Duntas LH, "Selenium and at-risk pregnancy," *Thyr Res*, 2020; 13(16). doi: 10.1186/s13044-020-00090-x

Grieger JA et al, "Maternal selenium, copper and zinc concentrations in early pregnancy, and the association with fertility," *Nutri*, 2019; 11(7): 1609. doi: 10.3390/nu11071609

Poormoosavi M et al, "The effect of follicular fluid selenium concentration on oocyte maturation in women with PCOS undergoing IVF/ICSI," *Int J Reprod Biomed*, 2021; 19(8): 689–98. doi: 10.18502/ijrm.v19i8.9616

66 Zinc

Garner TB et al, "Role of zinc in female reproduction," *Biol Reprod*, 2021; 104(5): 976–94. doi: 10.1093/biolre/ioab023

Prasad AS et al, "Zinc status and serum testosterone levels of healthy adults," *Nutr*, 1996; 12(5): 344–8; doi: 10.1016/s0899-9007(96)80058-x

Zhao J et al, "Zinc levels in seminal plasma and their correlation with male infertility," *Sci Rep*, 2016; 6: 22386. doi: 10.1038/srep22386

67 Iron

Chavarro JE et al, "Iron intake and risk of ovulatory infertility," *Obstet Gynecol*, 2006; 108(5): 1145–52. doi: 10.1097/01.AOG.0000238333.37423.ab

Diaz-Lopez A et al, "High and low haemoglobin levels in early pregnancy are associated to a higher risk of miscarriage,"

Nutr, 2021; 13(5): 1578. doi: 10.3390/nu13051578
Haider BA et al, "Anaemia, prenatal iron use, and risk of adverse pregnancy outcomes," *BMJ*, 2013; 346. doi: 10.1136/bmj.f3443

69 Choline and iodine
Korsmo HW, "Choline: exploring the growing science on its benefits for moms and babies," *Nutr*, 2019; 11(8). doi: 10.3390/nu11081823
Bath SC, "The effect of iodine deficiency during pregnancy on child development," *Nutr Soc*, 2019; 78(2), 150–60. doi:10.1017/S0029665118002835
Mills JL et al, "Delayed conception in women with low-urinary iodine concentrations," *Hum Reprod*, 2018; 33(3): 426–33. doi: 10.1093/humrep/dex379
Toloza F et al, "Consequences of severe iodine deficiency in pregnancy," *Front Endocrinol*, 2020; v11. doi: 10.3389/fendo.2020.00409

70–73 Supplements
Chavarro JE et al, "Use of multivitamins, intake of B vitamins and risk of ovulatory infertility," *Fertil Steril*, 89(3): 668–76. doi: 10.1016/j.fertnstert.2007.03.089
Majzoub A, Agarwal A, "Systematic review of antioxidant types and doses in male infertility: Benefits on semen parameters, advanced sperm function, assisted reproduction and live-birth rate," *Arab J Urol*, 2018; 16(1): 113–24. doi: 10.1016/j.aju.2017.11.013
House SH et al, "Folates, folic acid and preconception care," *JRSM Open*, 2021; 12(5): 2054270420980875. doi: 10.1177/2054270420980875
NHS, "Take a folic acid supplement" (online), 2020, www.nhs.uk/pregnancy/trying-for-a-baby/planning-your-pregnancy
UKTIS, "Use of methylfolate in pregnancy" (online), 2017. www.medicinesinpregnancy.org/bumps/monographs/use-of-methylfolate-in-pregnancy/
Akarsu S et al, "The association between coenzyme Q10 concentrations in follicular fluid with embryo morphokinetics and pregnancy rate in assisted reproductive techniques," *J Assist Reprod Genet*, 2017; 34(5): 599–605. doi: 10.1007/s10815-017-0882-x
Alahmar AT et al, "Coenzyme Q10 improves sperm parameters, oxidative stress markers and sperm DNA fragmentation in infertile patients with idiopathic oligoasthenozoospermia," *World J Mens Health*, 2021; 39(2). doi: 10.5534/wjmh.190145
Falsig A et al, "The influence of omega-3 fatty acids on semen quality markers," *Andrology*, 2019; doi: 10.1111/andr.12649

Agrawal A et al, "Comparison of metformin plus myoinositol vs metformin alone in PCOS women undergoing ovulation induction cycles," *Gynecol Endocrinol*, 2019; 35(6): 511–14. doi: 10.1080/09513590.2018.1549656
Lagana AS et al, "Myo-inositol supplementation reduces the amount of gonadotropins and length of ovarian stimulation in women undergoing IVF," *Arch Gynecol Obstet*, 2018; 298(4): 675–84. doi: 10.1007/s00404-018-4861-y
Merviel P et al, "Impact of myo-inositol treatment in women with polycystic ovary syndrome in assisted reproductive technologies," *Reprod Health*, 2021; 18(13). doi: 10.1186/s12978-021-01073-3
Roseff S, Montenegro M, "Inositol treatment for PCOS should be science-based and not arbitrary," *Int J Endocrinol*, 2020; 27; 2020: 6461254. doi: 10.1155/2020/6461254
Zheng X et al, "Inositol supplement improves clinical pregnancy rate in infertile women undergoing ovulation induction for ICSI or IVF-ET," *Medicine (Baltimore)*, 2017; 96(49). doi: 10.1097/MD.0000000000008842
Stanhiser J et al, "Omega-3 fatty acid supplementation and fecundability," *Hum Reprod*, 2022; 37(5): 1037–46. doi: 10.1093/humrep/deac027
Hashemi Z et al, "The effects of vitamin E supplementation on endometrial thickness, and gene expression of vascular endothelial growth factor and inflammatory cytokines among women with implantation failure," *J Matern Fetal Neonatal Med*, 2019; 32(1): 95–102. doi: 10.1080/14767058.2017.1372413
Cozzolino M et al, "Therapy with probiotics and synbiotics for polycystic ovarian syndrome," *Eur J Nutr*, 2020; 59(7): 2841–56. doi: 10.1007/s00394-020-02233-0
Lopez-Moreno A, Aguilera M, "Probiotics dietary supplementation for modulating endocrine and fertility microbiota dysbiosis," *Nutr*, 2020; 12(3): 757. doi: 10.3390/nu12030757

76–77 Exercise and fertility
Hakimi O, Cameron L, "Effect of exercise on ovulation," *Sports Med*, 2017; 47(8): 1555–67. doi: 10.1007/s40279-016-0669-8
Ibanez-Perez J et al, "An update on the implication of physical activity on semen quality," *Arch Gynecol Obstet*, 2019; 299(4): 901–21. doi: 10.1007/s00404-019-05045-8
Minas A et al, "Influence of physical activity on male fertility," *Andrologia*, 2022; 54(7). doi: 10.1111/and.14433
NHS, "Physical activity guidelines for adults aged 19 to 64" (online), 2021. www.

nhs.uk/live-well/exercise/exercise-guidelines/physical-activity-guidelines-for-adults-aged-19-to-64/
Shele G et al, "A systematic review of the effects of exercise on hormones in women with polycystic ovary syndrome," *J Funct Morphol Kinesiol*, 2020; 5(2): 35. doi: 10.3390/jfmk5020035
Vaamonde D et al, "Physically active men show better semen parameters and hormone values than sedentary men," *Eur J Appl Physiol*, 2012; 112(9): 3267–73. doi: 10.1007/s00421-011-2304-6

78–79 Sleep and fertility
Caetano G et al, "Impact of sleep on female and male reproductive functions," *Fertil Steril*, 2021; 115(3): 715–31. doi: 10.1016/j.fertnstert.2020.08.1429
Che T et al, "The association between sleep and metabolic syndrome," *Endocrinol*, 2021; 19. doi: 10.3389/fendo.2021.773646
Espino J et al, "Impact of melatonin supplementation in women with unexplained infertility undergoing fertility treatment," *Antioxidants*, 2019; 8(9): 338. doi: 10.3390/antiox8090338
Kloss JD et al, "Sleep, sleep disturbance and fertility in women," *Sleep Med Rev*, 2015; 22: 78–87. doi: 10.1016/j.smrv.2014.10.005

80–81 Stress and fertility
Clarke RN et al, "Relationship between psychological stress and semen quality among in-vitro fertilization patients," *Hum Reprod*, 1999; 14(3): 753–758. doi: 10.1093/humrep/14.3.753
Csemiczky G et al, "The influence of stress and state anxiety on the outcome of IVF-treatment," *Acta Obstet Gynecol Scand*, 2000; 79(2): 113–8. doi: 10.1034/j.1600-0412.2000.079002113.x
Dumbala S et al, "Effect of yoga on psychological distress among women receiving treatment for infertility," *Int J Yoga*, 2020; 13(2): 115–19. doi: 10.4103/ijoy.IJOY_34_19
Faramarzi M et al, "The effect of the cognitive behavioral therapy and pharmacotherapy on infertility stress," *Int J Fertil Steril*, 2013; 7(3): 199–206. PMID: 24520487
Palomba S et al, "Lifestyle and fertility: the influence of stress and quality of life on female fertility," *Reprod Biol Endocrinol*, 2018; 16(113). doi: 10.1186/s12958-018-0434-y
Purewal S et al, "Depression and state anxiety scores during assisted reproductive treatment are associated with outcome," *Reprod Biomed Online*, 2018; 36(6): 646–57. doi: 10.1016/j.rbmo.2018.03.010

About the author

Ro Huntriss is one of the UK's leading fertility dietitians with a bachelor's degree in Food Studies & Nutrition, a postgraduate diploma in Dietetics, and two master's degrees in Advanced Nutrition and Clinical Research. She's a researcher, published academic author in the field of fertility nutrition, and a clinician, with over 10 years experience working as a dietitian. Ro is also regularly featured in mainstream media outlets such as BBC, *Women's Health*, *Men's Health*, *Cosmopolitan*, and *HELLO!*.

A founding and existing committee member of the Maternal and Fertility Nutrition Specialist Group of the British Dietetic Association, Ro is passionate not just about helping women and men on their journey to conception and beyond, but also about educating fellow nutrition and health professionals on evidence-based ways in which nutrition and lifestyle can influence fertility so that more people can ultimately be supported on their fertility journeys.

Ro is an award-winning dietitian, having been titled Social Media Influencer 2022 by the British Dietetic Association for her work around fertility nutrition, and was awarded CN Magazine Community Nutrition Professional of the Year 2021.

As a huge advocate for the positive influence of diet and lifestyle on both male and female fertility, Ro regularly shares evidence-based content on her Instagram page @fertility.dietitian.uk and provides services through the wider Fertility Dietitian UK platform offering online courses, digital guides, and 1-2-1 consultations to her global audience. Discover Ro on www.fertilitydietitian.co.uk.

Author's acknowledgments

The author would like to thank Claire Attwood, ANutr, and Danielle Mulligan, RD, for their important contributions to this book and for being valued members of her team, and Kate Davies, RN, for her guidance.

Also, thanks to Claire Cross for her wisdom, patience, and talents in bringing this book to life. And thanks to Emma and Tom Forge for their beautiful layouts.

The author would also like to acknowledge her friends, Evelina, Anita, Mellissa, and Laura, for inspiring her journey into the world of fertility nutrition. She would like to applaud their strength, and also celebrate their successes on their own unique fertility journeys.

Publisher's acknowledgments

DK thank Claire Wedderburn-Maxwell for proofreading; Ginger Hultin for consulting on the US edition; and Hilary Bird for indexing.

Disclaimer

Neither the publisher nor the author is engaged in rendering professional advice or services to the individual reader. The recipes contained in this book have been created for the ingredients and techniques indicated and the ideas, procedures, and suggestions contained in this book are not intended as a substitute for consulting with your physician. The publisher is not responsible for your specific health or allergy needs that may require supervision. Neither the author nor the publisher shall be liable or responsible for any loss or damage allegedly arising from any information or suggestion in this book, including any adverse reactions you may have to the recipes contained in the book, whether you follow them as written or modify them to suit your personal dietary needs or tastes.

A note on gender identities

DK recognizes all gender identities, and acknowledges that the sex someone was assigned at birth based on their sexual organs may not align with their own gender identity. People may self-identify as any gender or no gender (including, but not limited to, that of a cis or trans woman, of a cis or trans man, or of a non-binary person).

As gender language, and its use in our society, evolves, the scientific and medical communities continue to reassess their own phrasing. Most of the studies referred to in this book use "women" to describe people whose sex was assigned as female at birth, and "men" to describe people whose sex was assigned as male at birth.

DK | Penguin Random House

Project Editor	Izzy Holton
Senior Designer	Barbara Zuniga
US Editor	Jennette ElNaggar
Jacket Designer	Amy Cox
Jacket Coordinator	Jasmin Lennie
Senior Production Editor	Tony Phipps
Senior Producer	Luca Bazzoli
DTP and Design Coordinator	Heather Blagden
Editorial Manager	Ruth O'Rourke
Design Manager	Marianne Markham
Editorial Director	Cara Armstrong
Art Director	Maxine Pedliham
Publishing Director	Katie Cowan
Senior Project Editor	Claire Cross
Senior Project Designers	Emma Forge and Tom Forge
Photographer	Luke Albert
Food and Prop Stylist	Libby Silbermann

First American Edition, 2023
Published in the United States by DK Publishing
1745 Broadway, 20th Floor, New York, NY 10019

Copyright © 2023 Dorling Kindersley Limited
DK, a Division of Penguin Random House LLC
23 24 25 26 27 10 9 8 7 6 5 4 3 2 1
001–333481–March/2023

A catalog record for this book
is available from the Library of Congress.
ISBN 978-0-7440-6966-2

Printed and bound in China

For the curious
www.dk.com

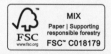

This book was made with Forest Stewardship Council™ certified paper—one small step in DK's commitment to a sustainable future. For more information go to www.dk.com/our-green-pledge